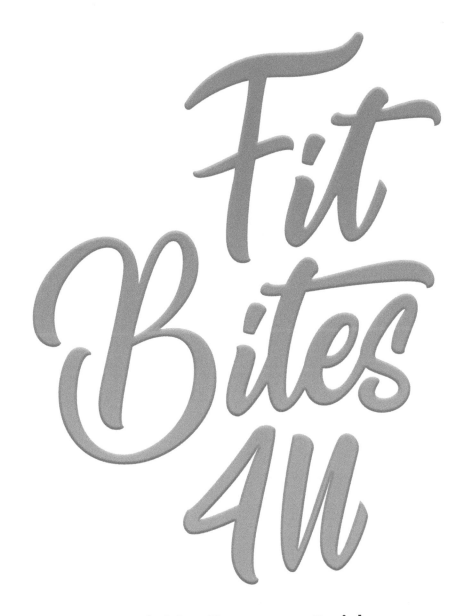

Fit Bites 4U

A No-Excuses Guide
To Healthy Meal Prep

BY NINA NYIRI

SUCCESS HAS NO DEADLINE, FAILURE IS NOT **FATAL**: IT IS THE **COURAGE TO MAKE CHANGE** AND COMMIT TO **SELF-CARE** THAT KEEPS US **GROWING**.

Contents

Introduction

Hey there! It's Nina here and I am beyond thrilled that you have purchased my first book. I am so blessed to have the opportunity to share my love for health and nutrition with you.

I know that starting a fitness journey can be extremely overwhelming because the media and food companies bombard us daily with the latest "trends" and newest "magic pill" that will get us the results we desire. I understand your frustrations because I've been in your shoes. I wasn't always "little miss fitness" and have had my fair share of epic disasters in the kitchen.

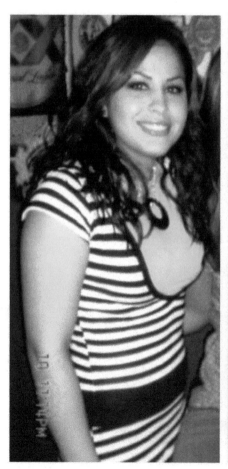 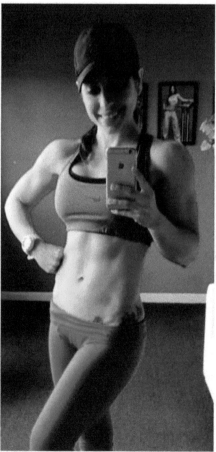

Up until the age of twenty-five, the extent of my cooking expertise included a microwave and ready-made meals. My freezer looked like I won the "Lean Cuisines" frozen food lottery and my refrigerator was bare to the bones - skim milk, cheese sticks, whole wheat bread and deli turkey. I was a frequenter at chinese buffets, I ate Texas-sized hunny buns and mocha frapps with extra chocolate chips were my jam. Yes, I ate like crap.

If you need more assurance that I was a terrible cook, my husband will tell you that when we first started dating, he would have preferred to throw a $50 bill in the oven because that's how much I wasted food. I've come light years and thankfully my husband didn't die of food poisoning along the way.

So if I can learn how to be confident in the kitchen, YOU CAN TOO!

As each day passes I'm understanding more and more how cooking nourishes our bodies on so many levels. When we cook we have total control over the quality and quantity of ingredients we are eating. But when eat out, or just fly by the seat of our pants, we relinquish that control.

We no longer know where our food is coming from, what kind of oils were used or even how our food was prepared. By cooking your own food, you *have control* and can make any adjustments according to your needs.

This book will not only provide you with easy and tasty recipes, but I will teach you how to kickstart your journey with simple nutrition tips and meal prep strategies. Failure is impossible because this journey is not about perfection. If you're ready to stop spinning in circles and wasting your time on another agonizing yo-yo diet that, let's make a change.

This book is definitely for you if:

- You've always been fearful of the kitchen and worried that making food is just too complicated.

- You've tried every diet on the block and nothing sticks.

- You are ready for change but don't know where to start.

Be on the lookout for "key" tips and habits that will accelerate your results!

"You can't build a great building on a weak foundation. You must have a solid foundation if you're going to have a strong superstructure."

- Gordon B. Hinckley

Nina's Basic Food Principles

When it comes to nutrition there is no one-size-fits-all plan.

After many years of research, self-experimentation, whoopsies and successes, I have found that these principles hold extreme value with body transformations. I think most of you reading this book not only want to make delicious recipes, but you'd like to see a better version of yourself in the mirror. These recommendations are suitable for a "healthy" individual — that's me politely saying that you should consult with your physician before you adopt any of these principles.

1. **Quality vs. Quantity.** This is an ongoing debate that will be highly dependent on the individual. So this is my opinion based on personal experience and results from clients. In the beginning stages of your journey, it is important to understand the impact quality foods have on your health. By creating awareness around healthier choices, you will be one step ahead of the game. After all, you are what you ate ate! And building the habit of choosing better foods is sustainable and doable long-term. It's important to understand that you can easily overeat healthy foods, so tracking your foods does have it's advantages. But to start, we are going to bring quality foods to the forefront. So what does that mean?

   - Choose humanely raised proteins and grass-fed cuts of meat. I would recommend applying a 90/10 rule when it comes to grass-fed vs. farm-raised meat. We take in animal's energy when eat it. So wouldn't you prefer to take in the energy of an animal that lived happily was treated humanely? To get organic and grass-fed meats delivered to your door, just visit butcherbox.com.

▪ Shop Organic as much as possible. Visit ewg.org to see the most-updated version of the "Clean Fifteen" and "Dirty Dozen" lists to help you make the best decisions when it comes to reducing your exposure to toxic pesticides. I recommend that you remove the skin unless you buy organic. Also, a majority of your condiments in jars or cans should be labeled as BPA Free and Organic.

2. **Eat real food.** This requires just a little bit of label reading. Anything "sciency" or looks like it belongs in an experiment shouldn't be in your body. So do your best to stick to minimally processed foods with the fewest ingredients. Remember the 80/20 rule -- it's what we eat consistently that matters the most.

3. **Sideline added sugar.** Sugar is the leading culprit behind cravings, uncontrollable appetite, unstable energy levels and an increase in belly fat. It also increases inflammation which has been linked to chronic diseases.

   ▪ Added sugars sneak into many of the foods we consume at restaurants, they are hiding in our drinks, salad dressings and cereal. Fact - a 12 oz. can of Coke has 40 grams of sugar -- the recommended daily allowance is 30 grams per day.

   ▪ Be on the lookout for ingredients ending in -ose and -ride (sucralose, dextrose, disaccharide, etc.). Rule of thumb, if sugar is listed as the first or second ingredient, this is not quality food.

4. **Reduce dairy consumption.** Dairy has also been linked to inflammation and can spike insulin. It can hold you back from losing weight and should be minimized within your dietary lifestyle. Ever wonder why you can't get rid of that mid-section fluff?

   ▪ If you're dairy intolerant, opt for non-dairy alternatives such as goat's or sheep's cheese, almond milk, coconut milk or hemp milk, etc.

- If you aren't sensitive to dairy, choose dairy products that are grass-fed and free of any added hormones.

5. **Eat your veggies.** We want food to keep us full right? Consuming veggies and complex carbs will keep your insulin in check due to their fibrous and nutrient-dense content.

    - Incorporate items from pages 32-33 on a regular basis to help control hunger and to keep you regular

    - Limit your consumption of simple carbs that lack fiber. They often leave you unsatisfied and intensify cravings. White or enriched breads, candy, sugary cereals and sugar-added yogurts should be considered "treats" not daily staples.

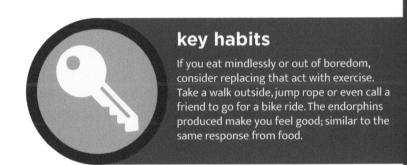

key habits

If you eat mindlessly or out of boredom, consider replacing that act with exercise. Take a walk outside, jump rope or even call a friend to go for a bike ride. The endorphins produced make you feel good; similar to the same response from food.

6. **Don't fear the fat.** Healthy fats are no longer the enemy — they definitely got a bad wrap over the past few decades. But it's time to toss the misconceptions and embrace their many benefits: Fats are essential for our body — full of antioxidants, supports brain health and metabolic functions and reduces inflammation.

    - Incorporate healthy fats such as avocado, coconut oil, extra-virgin olive oil, omega-3's, organic nuts and seeds, eggs, grass-fed beef and MCT oil.

    - Practice moderation with fats because they are calorie dense and you can easily overeat healthy foods.

    - The problem lies in the combination of highly processed fats and refined carbs which leads to excess calories, weight gain and many more health-related issues. This would be your average drive-thru order.

7. **Cycle your carbs.** Much like healthy fats, we demonize carbs to no end. They're not evil, but they should be consumed in moderation.

   - Incorporate a carb-cycling approach by adding complex carbs on training days and reducing them on your not-so-active days (Refer to page 32).

   - To maximize your training, time your carbs to be consumed around your training session; whether this be pre or post workout.

8. **Limit the frequency of your meals.** Before you knock it, try it. I used to eat 6 to 7 small meals per day and now I consume 2 larger meals with the occasional snack in between. Grazing throughout the day means insulin is running throughout your system all day long. And Insulin is a fat-storage hormone that works against the fat-burning Growth Hormone. When we eat every couple of hours, excess insulin is floating in our system and we simply don't have the ability to burn fat.

   - If you're constantly hungry (every 2 hours or so), first try consolidating your meals by adding more protein to your meal. This should leave you satisfied and save you time by not having to prepare an additional 3 to 4 meals.

- Give yourself at least 4 hours in between your meals to allow for proper digestion time. You never really get to tap into your stored fat if your body is trying to metabolize your previous meal(s).

9. **Take the judgement out of eating.** Anytime you feel guilty about eating, *this* is what will cause weight gain. Restriction of foods will likely lead to a vicious cycle of cravings, overeating and lack of control. It's just not worth it.

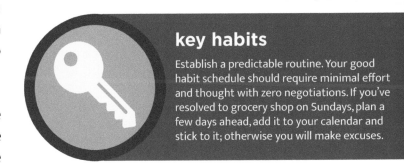

key habits

Establish a predictable routine. Your good habit schedule should require minimal effort and thought with zero negotiations. If you've resolved to grocery shop on Sundays, plan a few days ahead, add it to your calendar and stick to it; otherwise you will make excuses.

- Allow yourself quality "treats" in moderation during the week or when you feel you've earned them. Try to make your indulgence intentional.

- Avoid "cheat days" because in the long-run that may lead to a negative association with food and could be detrimental to your success.

10. **No extremes.** Extreme habits of any kind normally don't last. Why? Because they simply aren't sustainable for longevity.

- Eat moderately well, workout a few times per week, get enough sleep and repeat indefinitely.

- Remember that healthy eating is a combination of incorporating a balance of foods and having a healthy relationship with food.

The goal here isn't to choose just one principle and execute it with absolute perfection; the goal is to figure out which of these principles make you feel your best. Think about what foods and lifestyle choices really work for you.

Health-Boosting Foods

Too many times we forget the purpose of food and how it supports our daily living. We get so caught up in the temporary satisfaction with non-nutritious foods, which most often leaves us feeling unfulfilled, unhealthy and sick. Get a head start in building a healthier lifestyle by adding a few of these items to your daily routine.

Food	Brain Health	Gut Health	Heart Health	Immune Health	Skin Health	How to incorporate:
Bone Broth	✓	✓	✓	✓	✓	in a soup, with cauliflower rice, blend into smoothie
Coconut Oil	✓	✓	✓	✓	✓	cooking base, brush your teeth with it, as a moisturizer
Walnuts	✓	✓	✓	✓	✓	add to salads, on top of oatmeal, blend into smoothie
Dark Leafy Greens	✓	✓	✓	✓	✓	as a salad base, make a sandwich wrap, blend into smoothie
Avocado	✓	✓	✓		✓	with eggs, add to salads, sub for banana in smoothies
Extra Virgin Olive Oil	✓		✓	✓	✓	cooking base, sub for butter, salad dressing with lemon

Apple Cider Vinegar	✓	✓	✓	✓	in tea w/ honey, marinade with mustard, dilute w/ water & lemon
Blueberries	✓	✓	✓	✓	add to salads, with oatmeal, in a protein smoothie
Salmon	✓		✓		✓	bake or broil with olive oil and lemon
Whole Eggs	✓		✓	✓		hard-boiled, poached or omelette
Fermented Foods		✓		✓	✓	kombucha, saurkraut, pickeled vegetables, miso soup
Turmeric	✓		✓	✓		add to eggs, toss with roasted vegetables, blend into smoothie

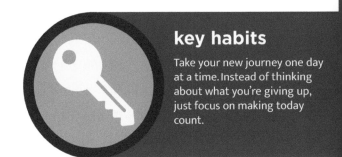

key habits

Take your new journey one day at a time. Instead of thinking about what you're giving up, just focus on making today count.

Simple Swaps

In order to build a healthy habit, we've got eliminate, replace or mitigate our old habits with new ones. The easiest way to start is by choosing your "most-used" non-nutritious items and gradually make your swaps as you see fit. A majority of these items are low-carb and dairy-free alternatives.

- Vegetable oil, Canola oil → Avocado Oil, Coconut Oil, Extra-Virgin Olive Oil
- Soy sauce → Coconut Secret Coconut aminos, Braggs liquid aminos
- Hellman's Mayo → Primal Kitchen Avocado Mayo
- Processed cheeses or cheese product → Nutritional yeast, Feta or Goat cheese
- Buttermilk, condensed milk → full-fat coconut milk or grass-fed heavy cream
- Cow's milk → Unsweetened Almond milk, Coconut, Hemp milk or Cashew milk
- Granulated sugar or Cane sugar → Swerve granulated sugar or Monkfruit sweetener
- Cornstarch → Arrowroot starch or Tapioca starch
- All-purpose, White flour → Almond, Coconut, Chickpea or Cassava Flour
- Margarine → Grass-fed butter, Ghee or Soy Free Vegan Butter
- White, Enriched Pasta → Banza or Tinkyada Brown Rice pasta
- White, Enriched Bread → Sweet Potato "Buns", Dave's Killer or Ezekial Sprouted Bread
- Banana (for smoothies) → Avocado or Sweet Potato (cooked)
- Maple syrup → Joseph's Lite Maple syrup or VitaFiber (prebiotic fiber sweetener)
- Chocolate chips → Lily's Stevia Chocolate Baking Chips or Enjoy Life Vegan Chips
- Ice Cream → Fro-yo, Sorbet, Non-dairy Ice Cream: So Delicious, Nada Moo, Coconut Bliss or Halo Top Dairy Free Ice Cream

Budget-Friendly Hacks

"I can't eat healthy because it's just way too expensive".

This was my mentality before I actually sat down and listed out ALL my food spending habits. Owning up to my daily food escapades made me realize how much I actually spent eating out. Talk about a reality check. Try this exercise now: Think about the trips you make to your local cafe, snack bar and favorite restaurant and write them down. These outings can accumulate to over $30 a day; adding up to $1,000 a month. Whoaaaaa Nelly!

There is definitely money to be saved by shopping purposefully! Just check out these tips:

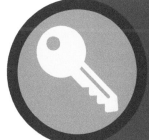

key habits

If you experience hunger pangs in the morning, drink water before you go straight for the breakfast sandwich. Keep in mind that you get in zero water as you sleep, so it's highly likely that what you're experiencing is actually dehydration and possibly a false sense of hunger. Water also helps your kidneys and liver to flush out the toxins that stress the body.

- Stick to your grocery list and never go hungry. If you're famished, you will likely make unnecessary purchases.

- Go to local farmers-markets. Not only is the food fresher, but local farmers tend to sell their organic fruits and vegetables at a much more reasonable cost vs. chain health food stores.

- Shop for produce that is in season. Eating seasonal foods is not only better for your health, but prices will be much more reasonable.

- Eat less meat. "Meatless Monday" is not only a great way to start your week, but you can also save money by consuming other forms of proteins like legumes, canned fish or eggs. Eggs are one the most inexpensive sources of protein.

- Stock up on sales. This is the best time to buy proteins in bulk because you can always store them in the freezer.

- Shop online. Don't let your busy schedule be an excuse to not eat healthier foods. Did you know many local grocery stores offer online shopping with delivery services? One of my absolute favorite online grocery stores is Thrive Market. You get awesome deals and can shop by dietary needs like Vegan, Paleo, Whole 30, etc. and they even support charitable companies.

- Learn to like leftovers. No sense in cooking every single night, because who has time for that?

  - Reheating methods: Use the microwave to speed up the process then finish off under the broiler or toaster oven; this will add a little crunch and stiffens the soggy.

  - Toss it over salad. Leftover proteins are the perfect addition to leafy greens.

  - Refrigerate or freeze your food within 2 hours of cooking. Store your food in BPA Free containers (I highly recommend glass, porcelain or stainless steel). Eat your leftovers within 2-4 days.

- Buy frozen vegetables. Always have a bag of _____ (you fill in the blank) as a back-up. I always keep a bag of frozen cauliflower rice readily available. Just steam, add butter/oil of choice and season with salt and pepper!

- Home-cooked Meal vs. Restaurant meal:

  Example 1
  Nina's Shortcut Chicken Caesar Salad (page 50)

Total: <$24 (4 meals = $6.00/meal)
VS. Caesar Salad at a chain restaurant will cost you $12-15/meal

Example 2
Nina's Blackened Salmon & Avocado Salsa (page 90)
Total: < $15 (2 meals = $7.50/meal)
VS. Small Salmon dinner at a chain restaurant will cost you $15-20

*Although organic produce and grass-fed meats are more expensive,
I think you'll find that they are still cheaper than eating out.*

Now that you have your game plan, on to Meal Prep!

Meal Prep 101

Cooking and food preparation is one of the highest acts of self-care you can engage in. And parents if you're cooking for your family -- this is the ultimate act of love. For most meal prep is an extremely daunting task because you don't where to begin, you don't how to make best use of your time, or you haven't been able to create habit of it. So, let's start with five basic tips to get you confident in the kitchen.

Simple Strategies

1. Think Differently

We are shifting the focus on what to eat rather than how much because quality foods will keep you satisfied and you will be able to lose body fat without obsessively counting calories. There's definitely a bigger picture beyond calories in and calories out. If counting calories was the answer, body image issues and obesity wouldn't be such common issues. Yes, calorie counting is necessary for awareness but it has the ability to cause unnecessary beat-yourself-down sessions.

2. Decide Your Menu

The way you pick your recipes can be simple. Firstly, all the recipes provided in this book are categorized by Training Day and Rest Day. All recipes are Gluten Free, Dairy-Free optional and can easily be customized to your dietary preferences.

Training Days. If you have regular workouts scheduled for the week, then it would be wise to choose one Training Day recipe per day. Training Day recipes include more complex carbs and fewer fats as compared to Rest Days. We implement complex carbs on training days to assist the body with recovery, to replenish depleted glycogen and to prevent fat loss plateaus. The Carb Cycling method will bring balance to your week, can help with sleep and you will always have carbs to look forward to.

Example Recipes for Training Days:

- Spaghetti Squash Casserole (page 66)
- Overnight Oats (page 116)

key habits

Add lemon to your water. Lemon is an acidic food which is very alkalizing to the body, it will boost your immune system and provide loads of antioxidants and minerals too.

Rest Days. You will likely have anywhere between 2-4 days of "Rest" during the week. These days can also be considered Active Recovery days. Rest is essential so that muscles can repair, rebuild and strengthen. Without sufficient rest time the body will continue to breakdown from intense exercise and risk of injury increases. We implement more healthy fats and vegetables on these days to help keep you satiated and to keep you in a fat burning zone. Rest days are comparable to a "Ketogenic" diet in that we include a moderate protein, high-fat and low-carb style of eating.

Example Recipes for Rest Days:

- Baked Ham & Eggs (page 110)
- Beef & Broccoli (page 62)
- These recipes can also be incorporated on Training days: just add a complex carb of choice.

A balanced approach to any dietary lifestyle is key simply because anything too extreme or restrictive is not sustainable for long periods of time. And the goal is to be successful long-term. So aim to eat intuitively and LISTEN to your body.

3. Create your Grocery List

Based on the recipes you choose for the week, add these items to your essentials. Print the recipe or take a screenshot of the recipe list.

Think about whether you want to make the amount it calls for or if you plan on doubling it for easy storage in the freezer. You will save more time shopping and you will less likely buy items that are unnecessary, so essentially you will be saving money.

Consider quick meals or grab-n-go items like these:

- Frozen Organic Veggies: always great for busy nights.
- Collagen or Plant-based Protein Powder: for those days when you know you are low on protein and need something quick.
- Hard-boiled eggs: great over a salad or a la carte. It's one of the most inexpensive sources of protein out there.
- Frozen Fish (preferably Wild-Caught): for those last-minute weeknight meals.
- Paleo Beef Sticks/Jerky: quick and reliable source of protein
- Uncured and Nitrate Free Deli Meats: great to roll, stuff and eat on-the-go
- BPA Free and Organic Canned foods: fish, olives, legumes
- Fermented pickles or sauerkraut
- Raw or unsalted nuts

4. Designate the Day

- Commit to a block of time for shopping and prep. This time is SO WORTH IT because you won't have to spend any additional time during the week worrying about your meals!
- The "Prep Time" indicated with each recipe will give you an idea of the total time required per recipe. So make sure to look at your recipes in advance.
- You are securing your week with the best choices for your body. It may seem expensive in the beginning, but think about how much you can potentially save on health care, doctors visits, medication and more. Just imagine how healthy you are going to be as you approach your 40's, 50's, 60's and beyond because of your choices NOW!
- You may find that you need to make more than one stop, so plan accordingly. I actually prefer to shop the night before I prep meals so I can just run home after work and get right to it! My usual route includes stops at Trader Joes, Publix (similar to H.E.B.), Whole Foods & Sprouts.

5. Kitchen Must-Haves

An artist can't create his masterpiece without the right brush! Check out this list of items you will need for meal prep and my recipes.

- Chef's Knife
- Glass Baking dishes
- 12-count Silicone Muffin Tin
- Food Processor
- Baking Sheet
- Non-stick skillet

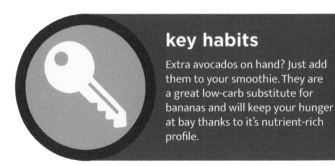

key habits

Extra avocados on hand? Just add them to your smoothie. They are a great low-carb substitute for bananas and will keep your hunger at bay thanks to it's nutrient-rich profile.

- Wooden spatula
- Circular baking pan
- Mixing bowls
- Crockpot/Instant Pot
- Cookie scoop

Not every week is going to be seamless. It's called LIFE and it happens. Just do your best to prep at least 75% of the month. Refer to this as a labor of love for yourself and your family.

Refrigerator & Freezer Items

PROTEINS

Pasture-raised Poultry:

- Chicken
- Turkey
- Eggs
- Duck
- Quail

Grass-fed Meats:

- Beef
- Bison
- Pork
- Venison
- Lamb
- Prosciutto

Wild-caught Fish:

- Alaskan Salmon, Smoked
- Bass
- Mackerel
- Shrimp
- Crab
- Lobster
- Scallops
- Tuna
- Calamari
- Sardines, Anchovies
- Oysters
- Mussels

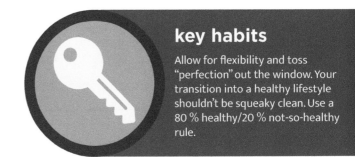

key habits

Allow for flexibility and toss "perfection" out the window. Your transition into a healthy lifestyle shouldn't be squeaky clean. Use a 80 % healthy/20 % not-so-healthy rule.

Plant-based:

- Organic Tempeh
- Sprouted or Hemp Tofu
- Veggie burgers (soy free)
- Pea protein powder
- Hemp protein powder
- Brown rice protein powder
- Nato

Dairy:

- Probiotic Yogurt or Kefir
- Goat cheese, Feta cheese (other raw cheeses from sheep's milk)

Uncured & Nitrate Free Deli-Meats:

- Turkey
- Roast Beef
- Bacon
- Ham

COMPLEX CARBOHYDRATES (Training Day):

(Training Day):

- Basmati, Jasmine or Brown Sprouted Rice
- Quinoa, Amaranth, Millet, Couscous
- Sprouted, Multigrain or Sourdough Breads
- Gluten free, Brown Rice Pastas
- Steel cut or Old-fashioned Oats
- All berries and fruits in season

VEGETABLES

Non-starchy (Everyday):

- leafy greens
- Spinach
- Cruciferous
- Brussel sprouts
- Broccoli
- Cauliflower
- Asparagus
- Mushrooms
- Green beans

- Cabbage
- Onions
- Shallots
- Zucchini
- Sauerkraut
- Summer squash
- Peppers
- Celery
- Cucumber
- Scallions

Starchy Root Vegetables (Training or Rest Days):

- Sweet potatoes, Yams
- Red or white potatoes
- Beans
- Legumes
- Lentils
- Carrots
- Green peas
- Spaghetti squash
- Butternut squash
- Beets
- Chickpeas

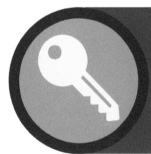

key habits

When you don't have time to cook, I suggest you look for a "farm-to-table" restaurant. You can still enjoy healthy food that tastes great.

SWEETENERS

- Stevia
- Monk Fruit
- Erythritol
- Xylitol

FLOURS

- Almond flour
- Coconut flour
- Cassava flour
- Hazelnut flour
- Arrowroot flour

CONDIMENTS

- ALL vinegars w/o added sugars
- ALL herbs and seasonings
- Mustard
- Tabasco
- Sriracha
- Fresh salsa
- Lemon, Lime
- Braggs
- Coconut Secret
- Primal Kitchen
- Tessemae's

FATS

For Cooking (high heat):

- Coconut oil
- Avocado oil
- MCT oil
- Beef Tallow
- Perilla oil
- Walnut oil
- Sesame Seed oil
- Macadamia oil
- Ghee
- Grass-fed butter

For Dressings (low heat):

- Extra Virgin Olive oil
- MCT oil
- Almond oil
- High-oleic Sunflower oil
- Truffle oil
- Macadamia Nut oil

For snacking/toppings:

- Avocado
- Olives
- Pistachios
- Almonds
- Walnuts
- Brazilian nuts
- Macadamia nuts
- Hazelnuts
- Almond butter
- Tahini
- Hemp hearts
- Flaxseeds/flaxseed meal

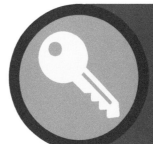

key habits

Leading by example can set the tone for your household. It may be difficult for your significant others to understand this new lifestyle, but don't give up on them.

Recipes

Poultry

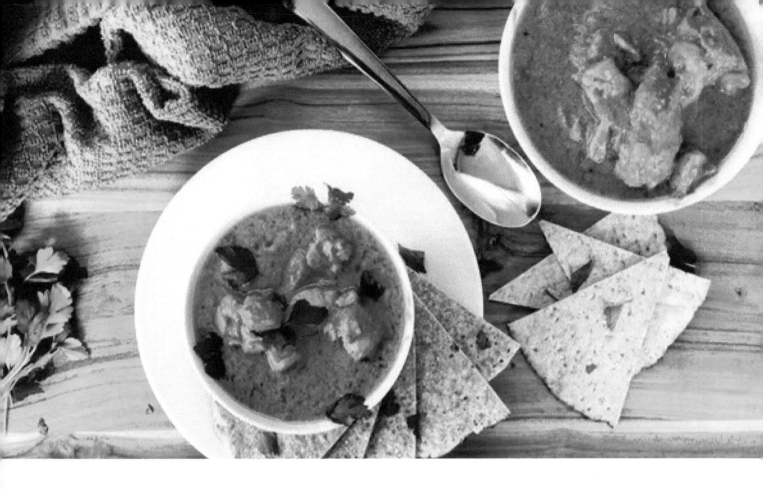

Instant Pot Thai Butter Chicken

Rest Day

Yield: 4 – 6 servings

Total Time: 15-20 minutes

Ingredients

....

- 4 tablespoons ghee or grassfed butter
- 1 pound chicken thighs boneless, skinless, cubed
- 1 medium white onion, diced
- 1 1/2 cups tomato sauce
- 1 1/2 cups canned coconut milk or heavy cream
- 1 tablespoon minced garlic

- 1 tablespoon fresh ginger, finely chopped
- 3 teaspoons garam masala
- 2 teaspoons chili powder
- 2 teaspoon turmeric
- 1 1/2 teaspoons cumin
- 1 teaspoon cayenne

Directions

....

1. Turn your Instant Pot to saute, medium, and add ghee or butter.
2. Once the butter has melted, add cubed chicken and diced onion. Cook for 5-6 minutes (just enough for chicken to cook just a touch on the outside).
3. Add the remaining ingredients into your Instant Pot and mix together well.
4. Put the lid on and close steam valve.
5. Set Instant Pot to manual, pressure for 5 minutes. If you have larger pieces of chicken, increase cooking time.
6. When the time goes off, carefully (with a towel) move the steam valve just slightly so steam comes out slowly. When there is no more steam, carefully lift the lid.
7. Allow the chicken to cool before serving. If you want the sauce to thicken a bit more, you can set the Instant Pot on saute (low) for just a few minutes.

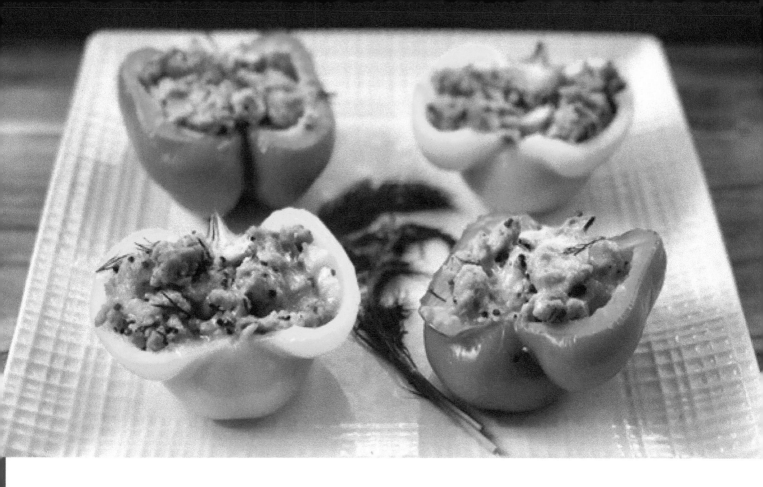

ITALIAN STUFFED PEPPERS

Rest Day

Yield: 2 servings

Total Time: 25-30 minutes

Ingredients

- 2 bell peppers, vertically sliced and seeded
- 1 tablespoon avocado oil
- 1/2 pound Italian chicken sausage or ground chicken
- 1/3 cup artichokes (marinated in oil), diced
- 2 small tomatoes, diced
- 1/2 cup quinoa, cooked

- Juice of 1 lemon
- 1 tablespoon minced garlic
- 2 teaspoons fresh dill, chopped
- 1/8 teaspoon pepper
- Pinch of sea salt
- 1/2 cup organic mozzarella or gouda cheese

Directions

1. Preheat oven to 350 F.
2. Place halved bell peppers on a baking sheet and cook for 15 minutes until just becoming tender. Remove and set aside. Set oven to Broil.
3. While the peppers cook, heat a non-stick skillet to medium and add avocado oil. Add the ground chicken and cook until no longer pink.
4. Stir in the remaining ingredients minus the cheese. Mix and turn the heat to simmer. Cook for another 3 – 5 minutes.
5. Spoon fill the meat mixture into each pepper, then top with the cheese.
6. Return the peppers to the oven and broil for 2 – 3 minutes until cheese has melted and peppers are golden brown.

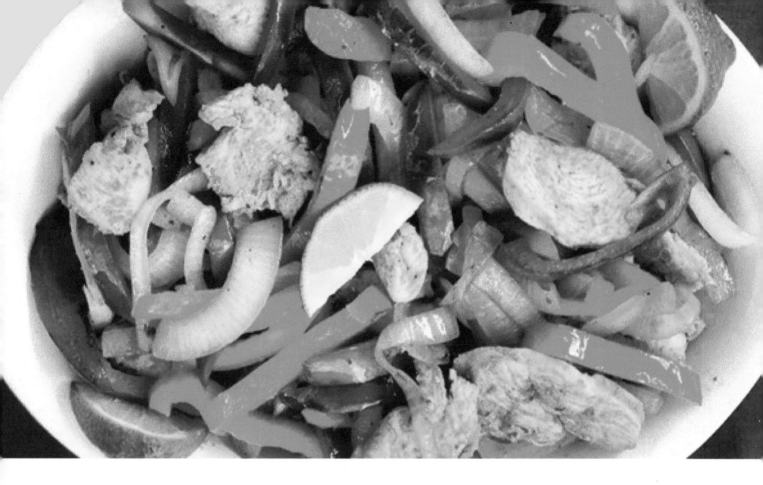

SKILLET FAJITAS

Rest Day

Yield: 4 servings

Total Time: 35-40 minutes

Ingredients

For the Chicken Fajitas:
- 1 pound boneless, skinless chicken breasts, cut into ¼" pieces
- 1 tablespoon avocado oil
- 1 teaspoon chili powder
- 1 teaspoon cumin
- 1 teaspoon chipotle chili powder
- ½ teaspoon hot sauce – optional
- 1 teaspoon garlic powder
- 1 teaspoon oregano
- ½ teaspoon sea salt
- ¼ teaspoon black pepper

For the Pepper and Onions:
- 1 white or red onion, sliced
- 1 red bell pepper, sliced
- 1 green bell pepper, sliced
- ½ teaspoon garlic powder
- ¼ teaspoon sea salt
- 1/8 teaspoon black pepper
- 2 tablespoons grassfed butter or ghee, divided
- Juice of 1 lime

For serving:
- Organic corn tortillas or lettuce wraps

Directions

1. In a large mixing bowl or Ziploc bag, combine the chicken fajita ingredients. Mix well and marinate for 10-15 minutes while you are prepping your veggies.
2. Preheat a large non-stick or cast iron skillet over medium-high heat and add 1 tablespoon butter.
3. When skillet is hot, add the peppers, onions, garlic powder, salt and pepper. Sauté the veggies for about 3-4 minutes until they have softened slightly. Remove the veggies and set aside on a plate.
4. Add another tablespoon of butter to the skillet and add the marinated chicken. Sauté until the chicken is cooked through and no longer pink.
5. Add the veggies back into the skillet along with the juice of 1 lime.
6. Sauté everything together for another minute. Serve over Siete tortillas or in a lettuce wrap.

Pro Tip: Use a ready-made taco seasoning to season the chicken.

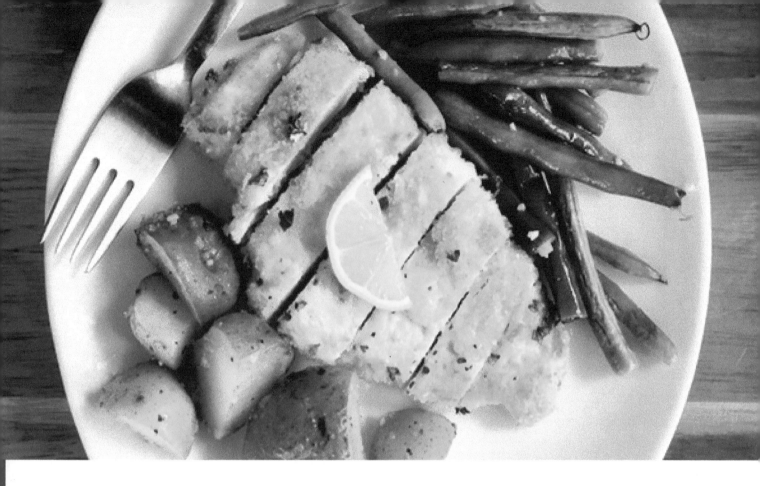

CRISPY ONE-PAN PARMESAN CHICKEN & VEGGIES

Training Day

Yield: 4 servings

Total Time: 35-40 minutes

Ingredients

For the Chicken:
- Olive oil cooking spray
- 4 skinless, boneless chicken breasts
- 1 large egg
- 1 teaspoon rice vinegar or juice of ½ lemon
- 2 teaspoons minced garlic
- 1 tables fresh parsley, chopped
- ½ teaspoon sea salt and pepper
- ½ cup gluten free panko or breadcrumbs

- 1/3 cup freshly grated parmesan cheese

For the veggies:
- 1 pound baby potatoes (medley), quartered
- ½ pound green beans, trimmed and halved
- 2 tablespoons grassfed butter or ghee, melted
- 2 teaspoons minced garlic
- Sea salt to taste

Directions

1. Preheat oven to 400F. Lightly grease a large baking sheet with cooking spray. Set aside.
2. In large bowl, combine the egg, vinegar/lemon juice, garlic, parsley, salt and pepper.
3. In another bowl, combine the breadcrumbs with the parmesan cheese.
4. Dip the chicken in the egg mixture, then dredge the chicken in the breadcrumb/parmesan mixture. Lightly press to evenly coat. Repeat for all breasts.
5. Place the coated chicken on to the baking sheet. Arrange the potatoes around the chicken in a single layer. Mix together the butter, 2 teaspoons garlic and salt to taste. Pour half of this mixture over the potatoes. Toss evenly to coat.
6. Bake for 15 minutes.
7. Remove baking sheet from the oven and gently flip each chicken breast. Move the potatoes side and make room for the green beans. Pour the remaining garlic butter sauce over the g and return to the oven on Broil (low) for another 10 minutes until the potatoes cooked more golden and crispy crust, add an additional 2 minutes' cook time on Broil (high)
8. Top with fresh parsley and serve immediately.

46

Pro Tip: For a kid-friendly version substitute chicken breasts for chicken tende

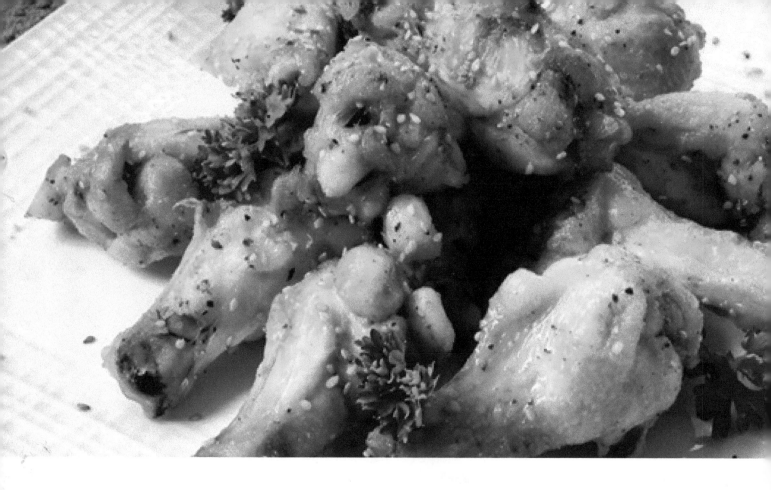

SESAME BAKED DRUMETTES

Rest Day

Yield: 4 – 6 servings

Total Time: 45-50 minutes

Ingredients

- 2 pounds chicken drummettes or wings
- 2 tablespoons avocado oil or olive oil
- 1 tablespoon toasted sesame oil
- Sea salt and pepper, to taste

- 2 tablespoons coconut aminos or Braggs aminos
- 1 teaspoon Red Boat fish sauce
- 1 tablespoon toasted sesame seeds

Directions

1. Preheat oven to 400 F.
2. Place drummettes in a large mixing bowl. Toss with avocado oil, sesame oil and season with salt and pepper. Mix well.
3. Arrange the drummettes on a large baking sheet on top of a wire rack.
4. Bake for 40-45 minutes until they are golden brown and crisp. For extra golden color and crispiness, cook on Broil (high) for 2-3 minutes.
5. In a small bowl, combine coconut aminos and fish sauce. Mix well and set aside.
6. Remove drummettes from oven and transfer into a bowl. Add the amino sauce and toss to coat. Add the sesame seeds and mix again.
7. Serve with cauliflower rice or with a side salad.

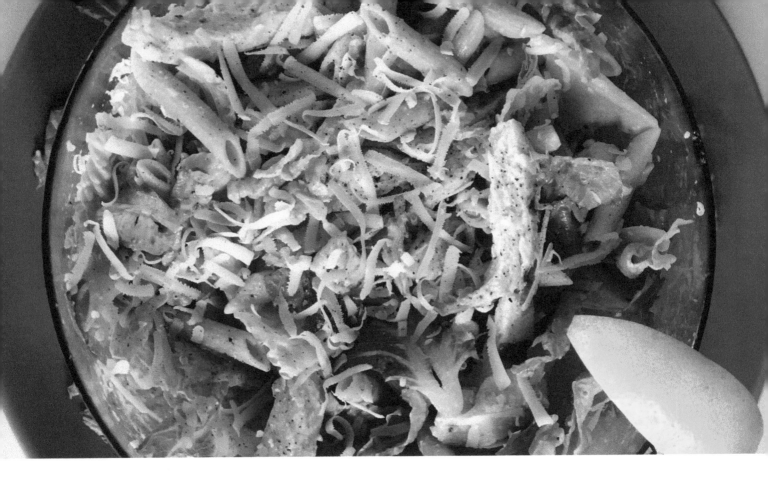

SHORTCUT CHICKEN CAESAR SALAD

Training Day

Yield: 4 servings

Total Time: 10 minutes

Ingredients

- 1 box *Banza* chickpea penne or brown rice penne
- 1 organic rotisserie chicken, de-boned
- 1 bag organic romaine lettuce
- 1/2 cup *Primal Kitchen* or *Tessemae's* Caesar Salad dressing
- Juice of 2 limes
- 1/2 cup shredded parmesan cheese
- Sea salt and pepper, to taste

Directions

1. Bring a large pot of water to a rolling boil. Cook pasta according to the package directions.
2. Drain the pasta in a colander under cold running water (this helps keep the pasta less-sticky).
3. Place the pasta in a large mixing bowl and add the remaining ingredients. Toss until coated evenly. Add more salt if necessary.

Pro Tip: For a rest day sub the pasta for more leafy greens and add diced avocado.

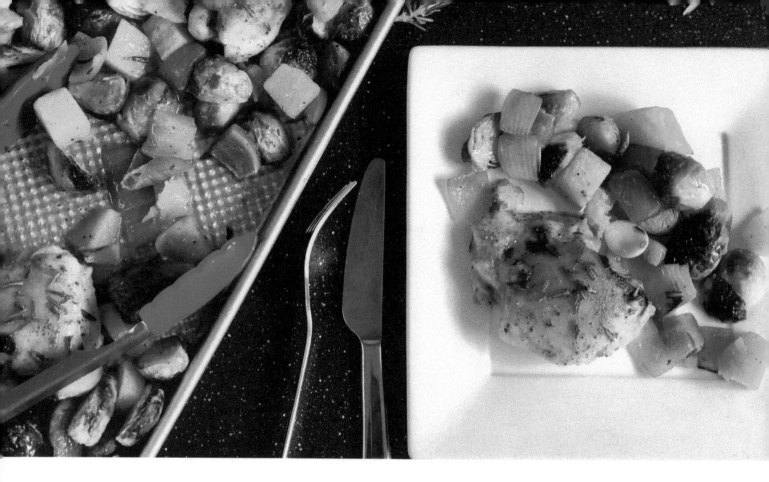

ROASTED ROSEMARY CHICKEN THIGHS WITH BRUSSEL SPROUTS & BUTTERNUT SQUASH

Rest Day

Yield: 4 servings

Total Time: 1 hour

Ingredients

- Olive oil cooking spray
- 1 to 1 ½ pounds boneless, skinless chicken thighs
- 3 tablespoons extra virgin olive or avocado oil, divided
- 1 teaspoon sea salt, divided
- 1 teaspoon pepper, divided

- 1 (12-ounce) packaged cubed butternut squash
- 1 pound brussel sprouts, trimmed and halved
- 1 red onion, sliced
- 10 whole garlic cloves
- 1 tablespoon honey
- 1 teaspoon dijon or whole grain mustard
- 2 tablespoons fresh rosemary, chopped

Directions

1. Preheat oven to 425F. Coat a large baking sheet with olive oil spray and place in the oven for 5 minutes.
2. In a mixing bowl, add the chicken thighs with 1 tablespoon oil, ½ teaspoon salt and ½ teaspoon pepper. Toss to evenly coat. Remove the baking sheet from oven and place the thighs on the sheet. Return the baking sheet to the oven for 8 to 10 minutes.
3. While the chicken is in the oven, combine the squash, brussel sprouts, onion, 1 tablespoon oil, ½ teaspoon salt and ½ teaspoon pepper in a mixing bowl. Toss until well combined. Set aside.
4. In a small mixing bowl, combine the garlic, honey and mustard. Whisk until well combined.
5. Remove the sheet from the oven and add the coated veggies around the thighs. Using a spoon, brush the honey mustard sauce onto the chicken.
6. Place the sheet back in the oven and bake for 15 minutes. At this time, sprinkle the rosemary over the chicken and return to the oven for another 10 to 15 minutes. Cook until chicken is done.

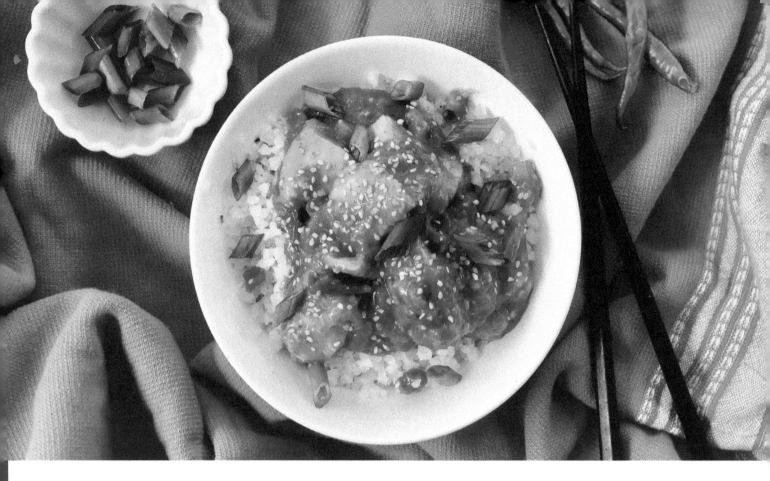

INSTANT POT SPICY
ASIAN CHICKEN

Training Day

Yield: 4 servings

Total Time: 35 – 40 minutes

Ingredients

- 1 – 1 1/2 pounds boneless, skinless chicken breast, diced into 1" pieces
- 3 tablespoons arrowroot starch
- 1/3 cup rice wine vinegar
- 1/2 cup coconut aminos or Braggs liquid aminos
- 2 tablespoons red chili peppers or red chili flakes, chopped
- 2 tablespoons tomato paste
- 1 tablespoon honey
- 1 tablespoon almond butter or cashew butter
- 2 tablespoons *Swerve* granulated sweetener – optional
- 2 tablespoons minced ginger
- 1/2 cup water
- 2 tablespoons avocado oil
- 1 tablespoon minced garlic

Toppings

- Green onions
- Sesame seeds

Directions

1. Place the chicken in large ziplock bag. Add the arrowroot powder to the chicken, and shake to coat so each piece is covered.
2. In a medium mixing bowl, combine the vinegar, aminos, chili pepper, tomato paste, honey, almond butter, sweetener, ginger and water. Whisk until somewhat smooth. Set aside.
3. Press the saute function on the Instant Pot. Once hot, add the avocado oil. Place garlic and chicken in the Instant Pot. Saute for 2-3 minutes, until the chicken is lightly browned on each side. Then press the cancel function. Pour the sauce on top of the chicken and mix until all pieces are evenly covered.
4. Secure the lid to your Instant Pot. Select the Manual function, and cook on high pressure for 8 minutes. Carefully use a manual quick release, and once steam is completely vented, open the lid.
5. Optional - If the sauce needs to be thicker, add in 1 additional tablespoon of arrowroot powder. Press the saute button cook for an additional 5 minutes.
6. Serve over basmati or jasmine rice and top with sesame seeds and green onions.

Pro Tip: For a rest day serve over cauliflower rice.

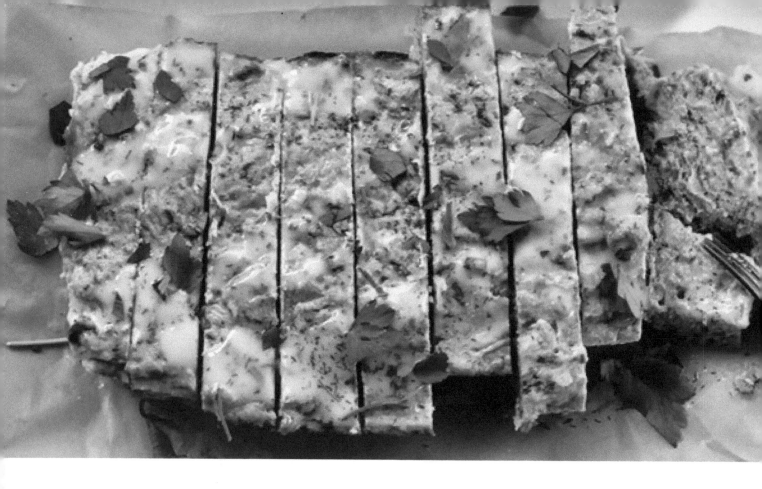

RANCH-STYLE MEATLOAF

Training Day

Yield: 4-6 servings

Total Time: 1 hour

Ingredients

- 2 tablespoons grassfed butter or ghee
- 2 tablespoons minced garlic
- 1 white onion, chopped
- 2 cups fresh spinach, chopped
- 2 large eggs
- 1 - 1 ½ pounds ground turkey or chicken

- ½ teaspoon sea salt
- ½ teaspoon pepper
- ¼ cup almond flour
- 2 tablespoons dijon or stone ground mustard
- 1 teaspoon of each: onion powder, garlic powder, smoked paprika, dried dill

Toppings

- *Primal Kitchen* or *Tessemae's Ranch dressing*

Directions

1. Preheat oven to 350F.
2. Heat the butter over medium heat in a non-stick skillet. Add the garlic and onions and saute until they have softened. Then add the spinach and cook until slightly wilted. Sprinkle with salt and pepper. Set aside and let cool.
3. In a large mixing bowl, combine the eggs, ground turkey, almond flour, salt, pepper, mustard and all seasonings. Transfer the spinach mixture into the bowl and mix using your hands or a wooden spatula.
4. Transfer meatloaf mixture to a greased loaf pan and cook for 45 to 50 minutes until juices run clear. Allow the meatloaf to cool before serving. Top with your ranch dressing and option to serve alongside skillet sweet potatoes.

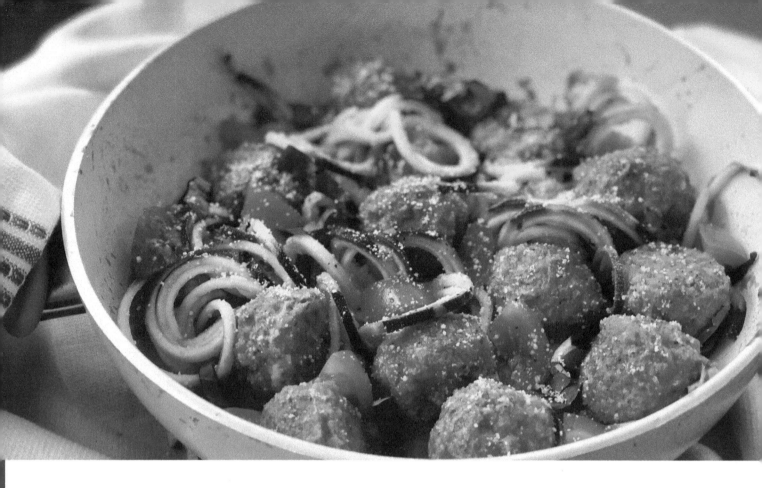

ITALIAN MEATBALLS
& ZOODLES

Rest Day

....

Yield: 4 servings

Total Time: 50-55 minutes

Ingredients

- 1 pound ground turkey, chicken, bison or pork
- 1/4 cup almond flour or gluten free breadcrumbs
- 1 tablespoon minced garlic
- 1 teaspoon oregano
- 1 teaspoon parsley
- 1 teaspoon Worcestershire sauce
- ½ teaspoon red chili flakes
- ½ teaspoon salt
- ¼ teaspoon pepper
- 1 large egg

Zoodle Ingredients

- 2 medium zucchinis, peeled or spiralized
- 2 cups organic marinara

Toppings

- Fresh basil, chopped
- Parmesan or nutritional yeast

Directions

1. Preheat oven to 400 F.
2. In a large bowl, mix all the ingredients until well combined. Using a melon ball scooper, shape mixture into 12-14 meatballs.
3. Place meatballs on a parchment-lined baking sheet and bake for 20-25 minutes. Baking time will vary depending on the size of your meatballs. Remove from the oven and set aside.
4. (Skillet option: using a non-stick skillet, add 1 tablespoon avocado oil and cook meatballs for 15-18 minutes, flipping every couple of minutes to ensure they cooked through and do not burn).
5. Once ready to serve, turn a non-stick skillet to medium heat and add the marinara. Once the sauce is warm, then add the meatballs. Gently coat the meatballs and then toss in the zoodles. Stir zoodles into the sauce and cook for 2 to 4 minutes until they soften to your liking.
6. Top with fresh basil and parmesan.

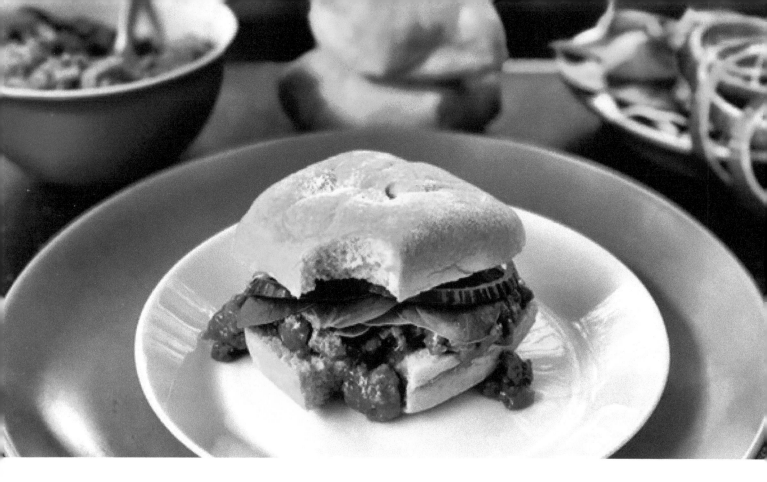

SIN-LESS SLOPPY JOE'S

Training Day

Yield: 4 servings

Total Time: 25-30 minutes

Ingredients

- 1 tablespoon avocado oil
- 1/2 medium white onion, diced
- 1 tablespoon minced garlic
- 1/4 teaspoon sea salt
- 1/4 teaspoon pepper
- 1/2 teaspoon cumin
- 1 pound ground beef, bison or turkey
- 2 tablespoons arrowroot starch
- 1/4 cup organic ketchup
- 2 teaspoons Worcestershire sauce
- 1 teaspoon Red Boat fish sauce
- 1/2 cup beef or chicken bone broth
- Buns of choice

Directions

1. Turn large non-stick skillet or cast iron to medium heat and add avocado oil.
2. Add diced onion and garlic, then season with salt and pepper. Saute until the onions are translucent and then add cumin.
3. Add the ground meat and break up the meat with a spatula, making sure there are no large pieces.
4. Once the meat is cooked through, add the arrowroot starch and stir until the starch has fully blended into the meat.
5. Add the ketchup, worcestershire, fish sauce and broth and mix well. Allow the sauce to come to a boil, then turn the heat down to simmer. Cook for 6-8 minutes until the sauce thickens (option to cover with a lid).
6. Remove the skillet from the heat and set to the side to cool. The sauce will continue to thicken as it rests.
7. Serve with a gluten free bun or alongside sweet potato fries.

Pro-tip: For a rest day use low carb Smart Buns by Smart Baking Company

Beef/Pork

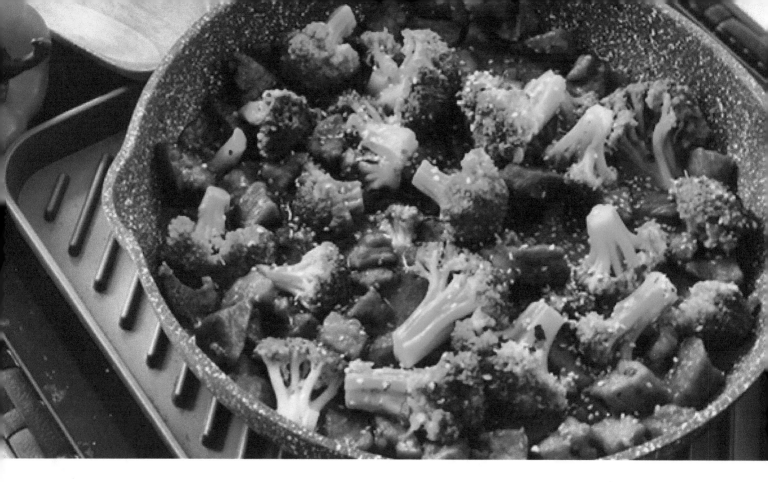

BEEF AND BROCCOLI

Rest Day

Yield: 4 servings

Total Time: 15 minutes

Ingredients

- 1 pound boneless sirloin steak tips or skirt steak
- 1 (16-ounce) frozen bag broccoli florets
- 1 tablespoon butter, ghee of avocado oil
- 2 tablespoons minced garlic
- 3 slices ginger, finely chopped
- Pinch of sea salt

Marinade

- 2 tablespoons coconut aminos or Braggs liquid aminos
- 1 tablespoon toasted sesame oil
- 1 teaspoon arrowroot powder
- 1/2 teaspoon sea salt
- 1/4 teaspoon pepper
- 1/4 teaspoon baking soda

Sauce

- 2 tablespoons coconut aminos or Braggs liquid aminos
- 1 tablespoon red boat fish sauce
- 2 teaspoons toasted sesame oil
- Pepper

Directions

1. Slice beef into 1/4-inch pieces. Add beef to a medium mixing bowl and combine the marinade ingredients. Mix well.
2. Cook the broccoli following the directions on the label. Set aside.
3. In a small mixing bowl, combine the sauce ingredients and mix well. Set aside
4. Turn a non-stick skillet or wok to medium heat and add butter or oil. Add garlic, ginger and pinch salt. Stir until fragrant (30 seconds - 1 minute).
5. Add the marinated beef to the skillet and cook until the beef is slightly charred on one side (3-4 minutes). Flip and cook until meat has darkened and has a crispy surface.
6. Add the cooked broccoli and sauce mixture to the skillet. Toss everything to combine.

Pro-tip: Save time by buying pre-sliced steak strips.

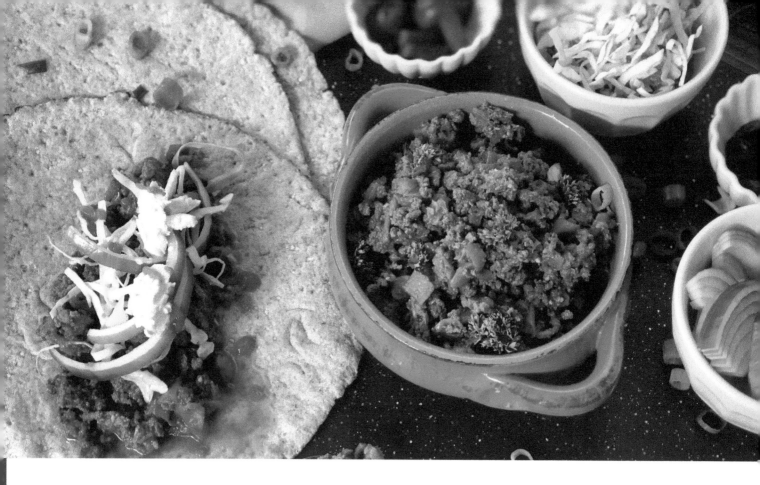

INSTANT POT TACO MEAT

Training Day

Yield: 8-12 servings

Total Time: 25-30 minutes

Ingredients

- 4 tablespoons avocado oil
- 1 red onion, diced
- 2 red bell peppers, diced
- 4 tablespoon minced garlic
- 2 teaspoons chili powder
- 2 teaspoons oregano
- 1 teaspoon salt

- 1 teaspoon dried basil
- 1 teaspoon smoked paprika
- 1 teasoon cumin
- 1/2 teaspoon cayenne
- 1/2 teaspoon chipotle powder
- 1/2 teaspoon pepper
- 2 pounds ground beef, bison, turkey or chicken

Directions

1. Turn your Instant Pot to saute and add the oil. Then add all the remaining ingredients minus the ground beef. Mix well and sauté for 5 to 6 minutes.
2. Add the ground meat and mix well. Cook until the ground meat is mostly brown. Put the lid on and close the steam valve. Set the Instant Pot o manual pressure for 10 minutes. Once the timer is up, allow the pressure to release naturally or carefully do the quick release.
3. Carefully open the lid and if the meat has released liquid you can press the Saute button to boil it off (optional).
4. Serve with lavash bread or naan.

Pro-tip: For a rest day serve over a salad or add it to your eggs.

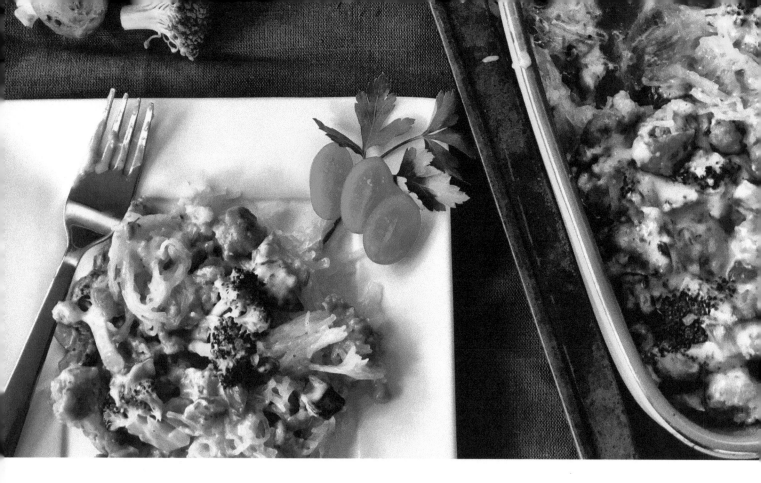

SPAGHETTI SQUASH CASSEROLE

Training Day

Yield: 4-6 servings

Total Time: 50 minutes – 1 hour

Ingredients

- 1 medium spaghetti squash
- 4 cups broccoli florets
- 1 pound sausage
- 2 cups button mushrooms, diced
- 1/4 cup arrowroot flour

- 2 tablespoons minced garlic
- 16-ounce canned coconut milk or heavy cream
- 1 teaspoon sea salt
- 1 teaspoon pepper

Directions

1. Preheat oven to 400 F.
2. Prepare Spaghetti Squash. See recipe for ""Spaghetti Squash Pad Thai" (page 108).
3. While the squash is cooking, start the sausage. Heat a large non-stick skillet over medium heat and add in the sausage. With a spatula break the sausage into pieces and stir occasionally, until browned and cooked through (about 8 minutes). Remove the cooked sausage from the skillet and set aside.
4. While the squash is cooling, turn the oven up to 425 F.
5. Heat the same skillet you cooked the sausage in over medium heat. Once hot, add mushrooms and cook until they begin to soften (about 2 minutes). Add in the arrowroot flour and minced garlic and mix well.
6. Add in the coconut milk and stir constantly for 2 minutes. To prevent flour clumps, be sure to mix well with a whisk. Allow the sauce to bubble and thicken and keep stirring to prevent the sauce from burning. After 2 minutes turn heat down to low and simmer. Add in the salt and pepper.
7. Lay the spaghetti squash "noodles" as the base in a medium casserole dish. Add the cooked sausage, broccoli, and creamy garlic sauce. Mix everything together well.
8. Bake the casserole for 15 minutes. Remove and allow to cool before serving.

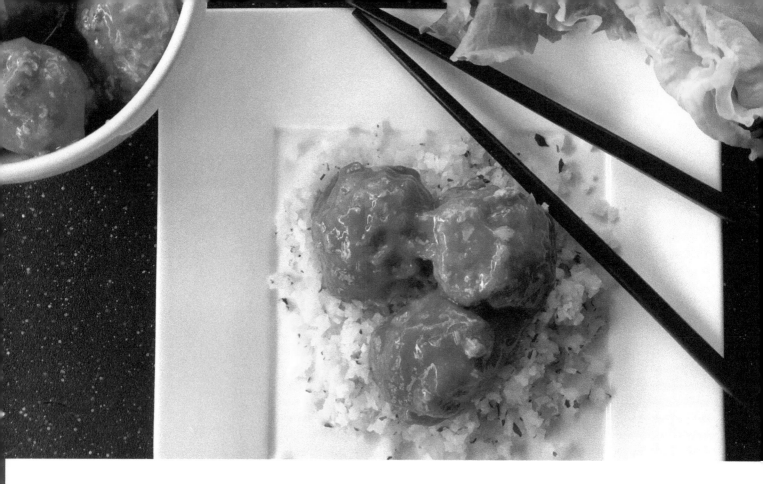

SWEET & SOUR PORK MEATBALLS

Rest Day

....

Yield: 8-12 servings

Total Time: 25-30 minutes

Meatball Ingredients

- 1 pound ground pork, beef, turkey or chicken
- 1 large egg
- 2 tablespoons almond flour
- 1/4 cup scallions, chopped
- 2 tablespoons coconut aminos or Braggs liquid aminos
- 1 teaspoon grated or minced ginger
- 1 teaspoon garlic paste

Sauce Ingredients

- ¼ cup tomato paste
- ¾ cup bone broth
- 3 tablespoons *Swerve* granulated sugar
- 2 tablespoons coconut vinegar
- 1/2 juice of lemon
- 1/2 teaspoon Red Boat fish sauce
- 1/2 teaspoon garlic paste
- 1/4 teaspoon grated or minced ginger
- 1/4 teaspoon guar gum (optional for thickening)

Directions

1. Preheat oven to 400F.
2. In a large mixing bowl, combine all the meatball ingredients and mix until well combined. Form 1 1/2-inch balls and place on coated or parchment-lined baking sheet. Bake for 20 minutes or until fully browned.
3. In a medium-sized saucepan, combine all the ingredients for the sauce and turn heat to medium. Stir frequently until the sauce comes to a rolling boil and reduce heat to simmer. Allow to simmer for 15-20 minutes, stirring occasionally. Option to add the guar gum at this point.
4. Once the meatballs are done, add them to the saucepan and gently turn to coat.
5. Serve over cauliflower rice or in lettuce wraps.

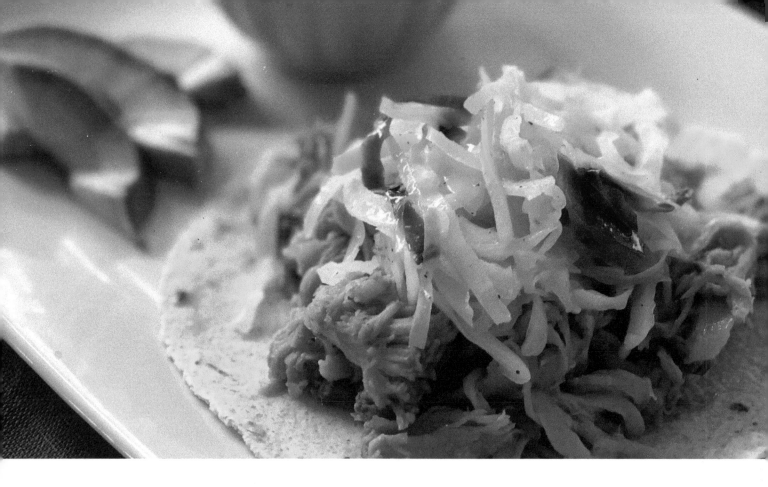

CROCKPOT MEXICAN PULLED PORK (CARNITAS)

Rest Day

Yield: 10-12 servings

Total Time: 4 hours

Ingredients

- 3 1/2 - 4 pounds pork shoulder
- 2 tablespoons cumin
- 2 tablespoons chili powder
- 2 tablespoons oregano
- 2 tablespoons granulated garlic

- 2 tablespoons powdered onion
- 2 tablespoon lime juice
- 2 cups beef or chicken bone broth
- 2 bay leaves
- Gluten free corn tortillas (for serving)

Toppings

- Avocado
- Salsa
- Red onions

- Green onions
- Sour cream

Directions

1. Optional - On a cutting board, after pork has been rinsed and dried, trim a majority of the excess fat (top layer) off. There is PLENTY of fat within the pork shoulder/butt to help keep the pork juicy and tender. You can also cut the pork into smaller pieces.
2. Optional - Line your crockpot.
3. Add pork to the crockpot and then season with all of the dry spices. With a spatula, rub the dry seasoning evenly onto the pork to make sure all pieces are evenly covered.
4. Add the lime juice and broth to the crockpot. Then add the bay leaves on top.
5. Set the crockpot on high for 4 hours.
6. After 4 hours, turn the crockpot off and allow the pork to cool for 10-15 minutes before serving.

71

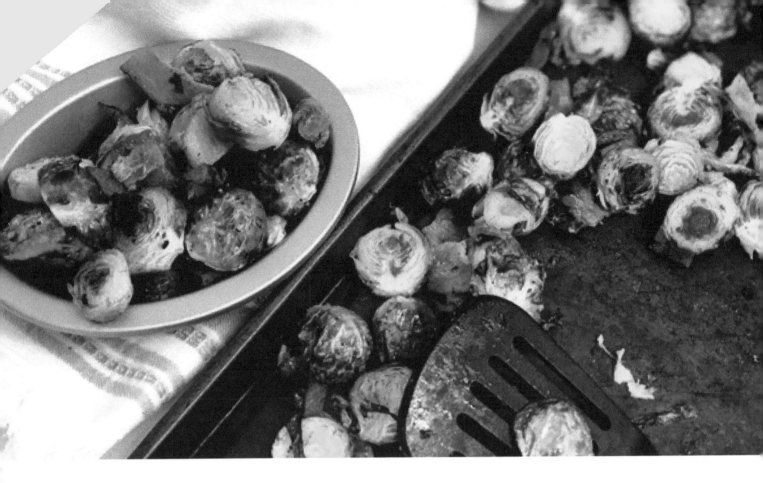

ROASTED GARLIC BRUSSEL SPROUTS & BACON

Training Day

Yield: 4 servings

Total Time: 20 minutes

Ingredients

- 1 pound Brussel sprouts, halved (may cut into thirds)
- 3 tablespoons avocado oil or extra virgin olive oil
- 1 tablespoon minced garlic
- 4 bacon slices, cooked and chopped
- 1/4 teaspoon sea salt
- 1/4 teaspoon pepper
- 2 tablespoons grated parmesan cheese – optional

Directions

1. Preheat oven to 400F.
2. Spread the sliced Brussel sprouts in a single layer on a baking sheet. Option to use aluminum foil or parchment paper. Roast for 18 – 20 minutes or until lightly golden brown and crispy.
3. While the sprouts are roasting, cook your bacon slices.
4. Optional - Remove the sprouts from the oven and top with parmesan cheese. Set oven to Broil and roast for 2 minutes.
5. Toss roasted sprouts with bacon and serve alongside a protein.

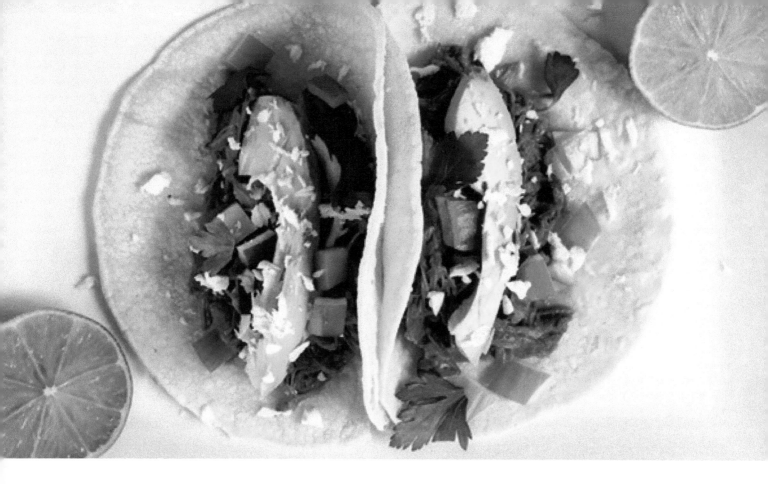

INSTANT POT BARBACOA

Rest Day

Yield: 8-10 servings

Total Time: 2 hours

Ingredients

- 2 ½ - 3 pounds rump roast or beef chuck roast
- sea salt to taste
- 3 tablespoons avocado oil or olive oil, divided
- 1 white onion, sliced thinly
- 3/4 cup beef or bone broth
- 2 - 3 chipotle peppers in adobo sauce (canned) + 1-2 teaspoons adobo sauce (preferred spice level)
- 2 tablespoons tomato paste
- 2 tablespoons apple cider vinegar
- 2 tablespoons coconut aminos
- 2 tablespoons minced garlic
- 2 tablespoons coconut sugar
- 1 teaspoon smoked paprika
- 1 teaspoon cumin
- 1 teaspoon oregano
- 2 bay leaves – optional

Toppings

- Red onions
- Avocado
- Cilantro
- Hot sauce
- Lime wedges

Directions

1. Cut roast into 4-5 hunks of meat. Season generously with sea salt.
2. Press the "saute" button on the Instant Pot.
3. Add the oil to the bottom of the pot. Sear the meat in batches until all of the meat is browned on all sides. (3-4 minutes per side). Set the meat on a plate until all meat is browned.
4. When all the meat is set aside, add 1 more tablespoon of oil to the Instant Pot and add the onions. Saute the onions for 3-4 minutes.
5. Hit "cancel" and nestle the meat back into the pot all in one layer (even if it's a tight fit).
6. In a medium mixing bowl, combine the broth, chipotle peppers, tomato paste, apple cider vinegar, coconut aminos, minced garlic, coconut sugar, smoked paprika, cumin and oregano. Whisk until well combined.
7. Pour the sauce over the meat and option to throw in the bay leafs. Cover and lock the lid.
8. Hit "manual" and set the timer for 90 minutes.
9. When cook time is complete, press "cancel" and carefully release the pressure manually. Once the steam is completely vented, open the lid.
10. Using tongs. transfer the meat to a baking sheet. This will help the juices not get everywhere. Use forks to shred the meat.
11. Serve immediately on corn tortillas or place in meat back into the juices until ready to serve.

Pro-tip: If using a crockpot, brown meat in a skillet then transfer to slow cooker. Add remaining ingredients and cook on low for 8-10 hours.

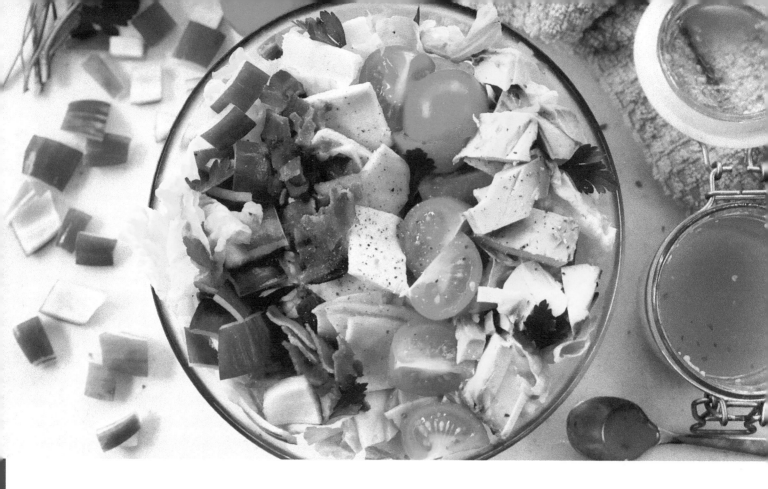

BLT SALAD & GARLIC VINAIGRETTE

Rest Day

....

Yield: 1 serving (4 servings for dressing)

Total Time: 5 minutes

Dressing Ingredients

- 2 tablespoons apple cider vinegar
- 4 – 5 tablespoons extra virgin olive oil
- 2 teaspoons minced garlic

- 1 packet Monk Fruit in the Raw or 1 teaspoon stevia powder
- 1/2 teaspoon sea salt

Salad Ingredients

- 2 cups romaine or spinach, chopped
- 2 ounces turkey slices
- 1/2 cup cherry tomatoes
- 1/2 avocado

- 2 slices bacon, cooked and chopped
- 1/2 cup cucumber, chopped
- 1/4 red onion, chopped

Directions

1. For the dressing, add all the ingredients in a jar with a tightly-fitted lid.
2. Close the lid tight and shake vigorously.
3. Prepare you salad ingredients and top with 2 tablespoons of dressing.
4. Top with fresh parsley and pepper.

Pro-tip: For additional fat add hard-boiled eggs or avocado.

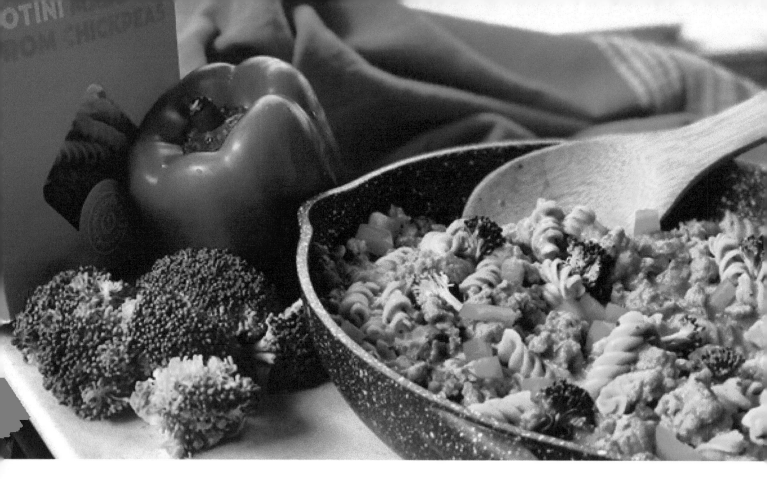

HEART HEALTHY
HAMBURGER HELPER

Training Day

Yield: 4-5 servings

Total Time: 25-30 minutes

Ingredients

- 1 tablespoon avocado oil
- 1 pound ground beef, bison, pork or turkey
- 1 teaspoon smoked paprika
- 1 teaspoon oregano
- 1 teaspoon parsley
- 1 teaspoon garlic powder
- 1 teaspoon onion powder
- 1/2 teaspoon chili powder
- 1/2 teaspoon sea salt

- 2 tablespoons tomato paste
- 1 1/2 cups almond milk or coconut milk
- 1 cup beef bone broth
- 2 teaspoons Worcestershire sauce
- 4 ounces *Banza* Rotini or brown rice pasta
- 1 tablespoon arrowroot starch
- 1/2 cup sharp cheddar cheese - optional

Directions

1. Heat a large non-stick skillet or cast iron on medium and add avocado oil.
2. Add ground meat and cook until fully browned.
3. Add paprika, oregano, parsley, garlic powder, onion powder, chili powder and sea salt. Mix until well combined.
4. Add tomato paste, milk, broth, Worcestershire and pasta. Gently mix until well combined. Reduce heat to simmer and cover. Simmer for 10 – 15 minutes until the noodles are to your preference.
5. Remove the skillet from the heat and add the arrowroot starch. Stir until starch has fully dissolved. Then add the cheese – optional.

Pro-tip: Keep it dairy free by adding Follow Your Heart parmesan.

Seafood

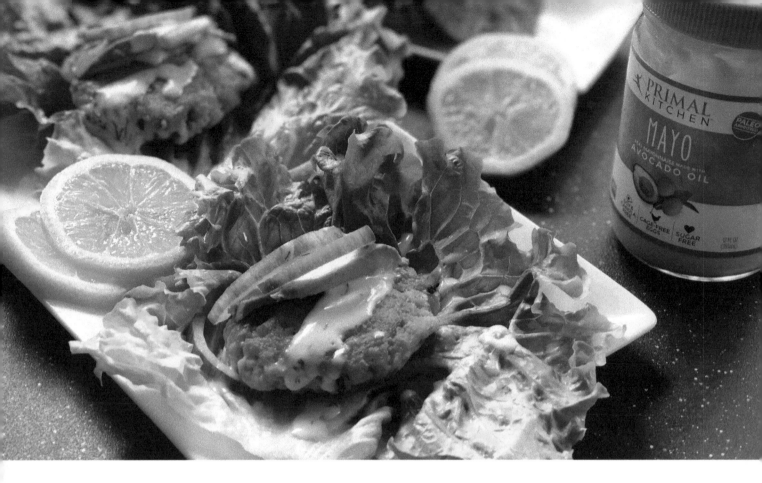

SALMON BURGER PATTIES

Rest Day

···

Yield: 4 servings

Total Time: 15-20 minutes

Ingredients

- 3 (6-ounce) cans wild Alaskan salmon, drained
- 2 ounces smoked salmon pieces, chopped
- 1/4 cup almond flour
- 1 large egg
- 3 tablespoons *Primal Kitchen* Mayo, divided
- 2 tablespoons green onions, chopped
- 1 tablespoon + teaspoon lemon juice, divided
- 1 teaspoon salt
- 1-2 tablespoons coconut oil or ghee
- 1 tsp fresh dill, chopped
- Lettuce leaves (for serving)

Toppings

- Avocado
- Red onions

Directions

1. In a medium bowl, combine salmon, almond flour, egg, 2 tablespoons mayo, green onions, 1 teaspoon lemon juice and salt. Best to use your hands to combine. Using a ¼ cup measurer, form 8 patties.
2. Using a cast iron or nonstick skillet, turn heat to medium high and add oil or ghee. Add the patties and cook for about 3 minutes and carefully flip with a spatula. Continue to cook for another 2-3 minutes until light golden brown on each side.
3. When ready to serve, option to make a dill sauce. Combine 1 tablespoon mayo, 1 tablespoon lime juice and dill. Stir well to combine.
4. Serve burger patties over lettuce leaves and top with avocado and red onions.

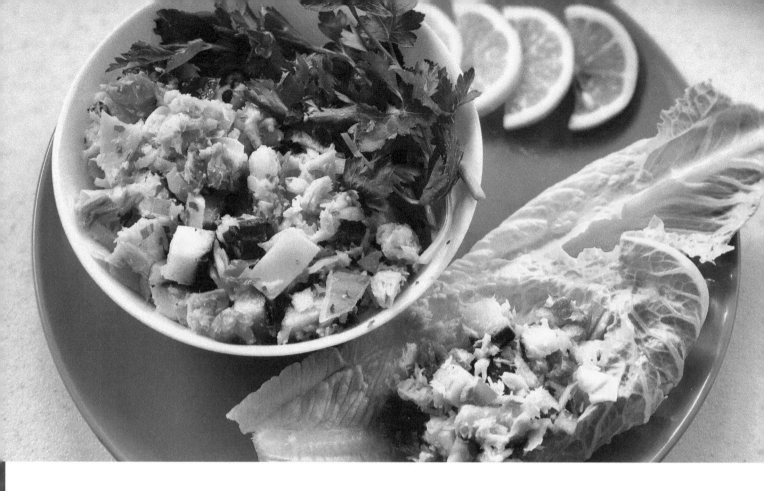

MEDITERRANEAN TUNA SALAD

Rest Day

Yield: 2 servings

Total Time: 10 minutes

Ingredients

- 2 (4.5-ounce) cans wild albacore tuna in water, drained
- ½ cup artichokes marinated in oil, chopped
- ½ cup sun-dried tomatoes, chopped
- ½ cup cucumber, chopped and seeds removed
- ¼ medium red onion, chopped
- Zest of 1 lemon
- Juice of ½ lemon
- 3 tablespoons extra virgin olive oil
- 2 tablespoons fresh basil, chopped
- 1 teaspoon minced garlic
- ¼ teaspoon sea salt
- 1/8 teaspoon pepper
- Pinch of red chili flakes

Directions

1. In a large mixing bowl, add the tuna and break it up into bite-size pieces with a fork.
2. Add all of the ingredients, mix well and serve!

Pro-tip: Add a heart-healthy dose of Omega 3's by swapping tuna for wild-caught salmon.

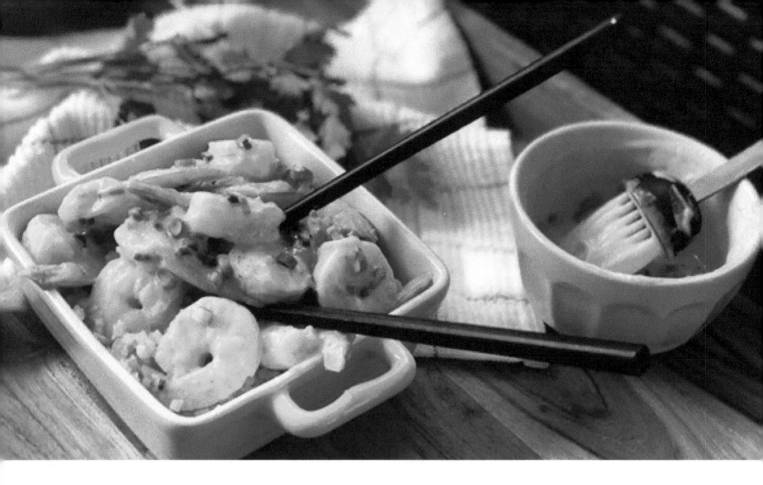

BAKED BANG BANG SHRIMP

Rest Day

Yield: 2 servings

Total Time: 10-15 minutes

Ingredients

- 2 tablespoons *Kite Hill* plain almond milk yogurt or plain greek yogurt
- 2 tablespoons green onions, chopped
- 1 tablespoons Franks hot sweet chili sauce
- 1 - 2 teaspoons sriracha - optional
- ½ pound shrimp, cooked or uncooked shrimp (peeled and deveined)

Directions

1. In a small mixing bowl, combine the yogurt, green onions, sweet chili sauce and sriracha. Whisk until well combined. For a thicker sauce, add 1 tablespoon Primal Kitchen mayo.
2. For raw shrimp: place shrimp on skewers and bake for 5 - 8 minutes on each side until no longer see through.
3. For pre-cooked shrimp: place shrimp on skewers and bake for 5 - 10 minutes (total) until fully warmed through.
4. Brush the skewers with the sauce on both sides. Serve immediately over cauliflower rice.

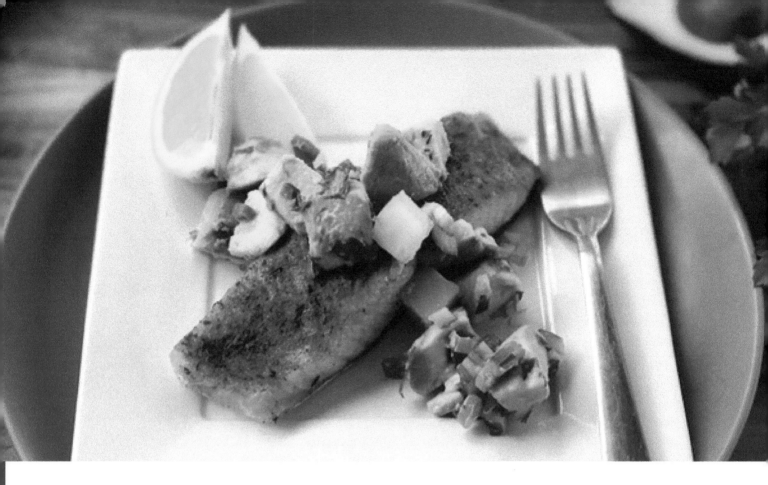

BLACKENED SALMON
& AVOCADO SALSA

Yield: 2 servings

Total Time: 10 minutes

Ingredients

- 2 (6-ounce) Wild Alaskan salmon fillets (skin optional)
- 2 teaspoons cajun or creole seasoning, divided
- 1 avocado, diced
- ½ cup cucumber, diced and seeded (optional)
- 2 tablespoons green onion, chopped
- 1 tablespoon fresh parsley, chopped
- 2 teaspoons lemon juice
- Sea salt to taste

Directions

1. Preheat broiler (high) with oven rack 6 inches from the heat. Place fillets, skin side down a foil-lined baking sheet. Add cajun/creole seasoning and pat down evenly.
2. Broil to desired degree of doneness, 8 to 10 minutes. (Option to cook on the stovetop: Heat 1 tablespoon avocado oil in a cast-iron skillet over medium-high heat. Add the seasoned salmon and cook until golden brown to slightly blackened before flipping. Repeat and cook to desired doneness).
3. While the salmon is baking, add the remaining ingredients to a mixing bowl. Combine and set aside.
4. Serve salmon with avocado salsa.

Pro-tip: Always keep frozen and wild-caught salmon fillets on hand for last-minute meals.

Meatless

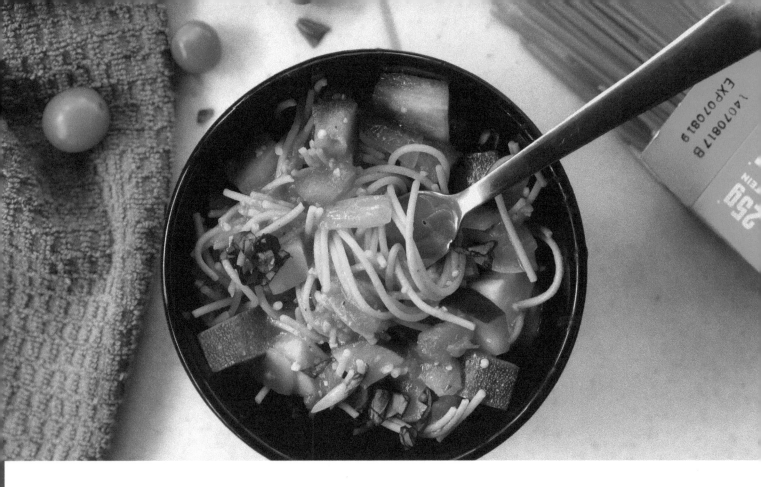

VEGAN RATATOUILLE

Training Day

Yield: *4 servings*

Total Time: *25 - 30 minutes*

Ingredients

- 1 tablespoon avocado oil
- 1 small onion, diced
- 2 tablespoon minced garlic
- 1/2 eggplant, diced
- 1 medium zucchini, diced
- 1 red or orange bell pepper, diced
- 1 (14.5-ounce) can diced tomatoes, drained
- 1 teaspoon tomato paste
- 1 teaspoon balsamic vinegar
- 2 cups boiled water
- 4-5 oz. *Banza* chickpea spaghetti or brown rice spaghetti
- Sea salt and pepper to taste

Toppings

- Fresh basil
- Nutritional yeast or dairy free parmesan

Directions

1. Add avocado oil to non-stick skillet and bring to medium heat. Add the onions, garlic, eggplant, zucchini and pepper. Sauté for a few minutes on medium-high heat until lightly browned.
2. Add the drained tomatoes, tomato paste, balsamic vinegar and water. Gently stir mixing well. Then add the spaghetti. Bring to a boil then simmer for 10 minutes until the pasta is cooked and the sauce has thickened.
3. Once ready to serve, add chopped basil, nutritional yeast salt and pepper.

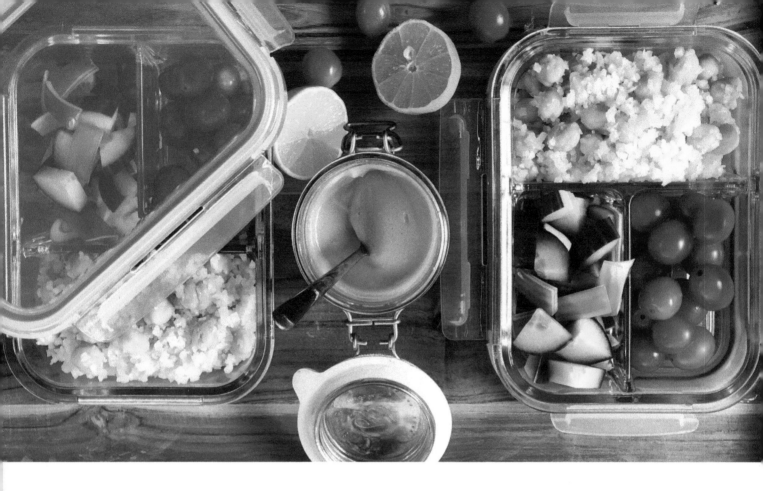

CHICKPEA BOWL W/TAHINI DRESSING

Training Day

Yield: 2 servings

Total Time: 10-15 minutes

Ingredients

- 1 cup cooked chickpeas
- 2 cups riced cauliflower
- 1/4 teaspoon sea salt
- 1 medium cucumber
- ½ pint cherry tomatoes
- 1 small red onion

- 4 ounces cubed feta (200g)
- 1 tablespoon lemon juice
- 1 tablespoon tahini
- 1 teaspoon honey
- 4 tablespoons extra virgin olive oil
- sea salt & black pepper to taste

Directions

1. Sauté cauliflower rice in non-stick skillet over medium heat and add salt. Cook until it is to your desired texture.
2. In the meantime, wash and cut vegetables and divide all ingredients in 4 parts and add to 4 large bowls.
3. Prepare salad dressing by mixing lemon juice, tahini, honey and olive oil in an airtight container and shake until well combined.
4. Once cauliflower has cooled, then divide into 4 parts and add to bowls
5. Immediately refrigerate and take 1 bowl to work with 1/4 of the dressing. Give the dressing a shake before adding to bowl.

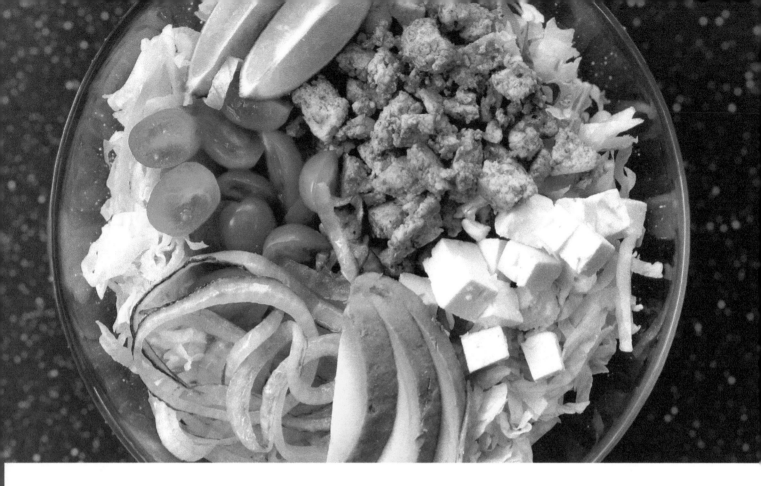

VEGAN TOFU TACO BOWL

Rest Day

Yield: 2-3 servings

Total Time: 10-15 minutes

Ingredients

- 14 ounces extra firm tofu
- 2 Tablespoons avocado oil
- 1 teaspoon cumin
- 1 teaspoon chili powder
- 1 teaspoon smoked paprika
- 1 teaspoon garlic powder
- 1/2 teaspoon sea salt
- 1/2 teaspoon pepper
- Pinch of cayenne

Toppings

- Shredded lettuce, spinach or kale
- Avocado or guacamole
- Grilled white or red onion
- Tomatoes or salsa

Directions

1. Remove as much excess liquid and moisture from the tofu by placing the tofu block on paper towels. Put another layer of towels on top of the tofu. Put a plate or a cutting board on top of the paper towels and then weigh it down with heavy books or cans.
2. In a large skillet, heat oil to medium and add the block of tofu. Use spatula to break up the tofu into small pieces. Add seasonings and continue stirring until all of the tofu is seasoned.
3. Cook for 8-10 minutes, until tofu is heated throughout.
4. Prep your toppings and serve!

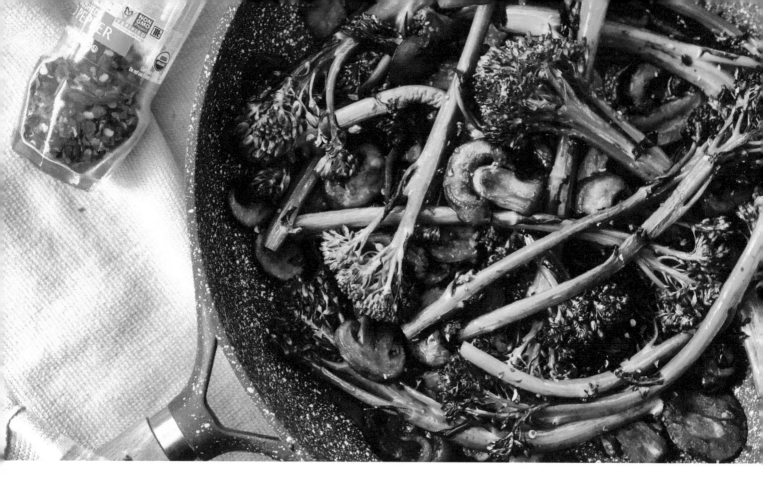

BALSAMIC GLAZED
BROCCOLINI AND MUSHROOMS

Rest Day/Training Day

Yield: 3 – 4 servings

Total Time: 25-30 minutes

Ingredients

- 1 pound broccolini
- 2 tablespoons avocado oil, divided
- 1 large shallot, thinly sliced
- ½ pound baby portobello or cremini mushrooms
- 1 teaspoon grassfed butter or ghee

- 2 tablespoons bone broth or vegetable broth
- 2 tablespoons balsamic vinegar
- ¼ teaspoon sea salt
- 1/8 teaspoon pepper
- Red chili flakes

Directions

1. Preheat oven to 400 F.
2. Place the broccolini a baking sheet and add drizzle 1 tablespoon avocado oil. Lightly sprinkle salt and pepper and toss to evenly coat. Spread the broccolini on the baking sheet in one layer.
3. Roast the broccolini for 12 – 15 minutes or until tender. Remove from the oven and set aside.
4. While the broccolini is roasting, add 1 tablespoon avocado oil to medium non-stick skillet. Turn heat to medium and add the shallots. Sauté for a few minutes until they have softened.
5. Add in the mushrooms and turn the heat to medium-high. Sauté the mushrooms for 5 – 8 minutes. After the moisture from the mushrooms evaporates, add butter and stir.
6. Then add the broth and balsamic vinegar. Continue to sauté for another 3 – 5 minutes until the liquid cooks down.
7. Once ready to serve, plate the broccolini and top with mushrooms and a pinch of red chili flakes.

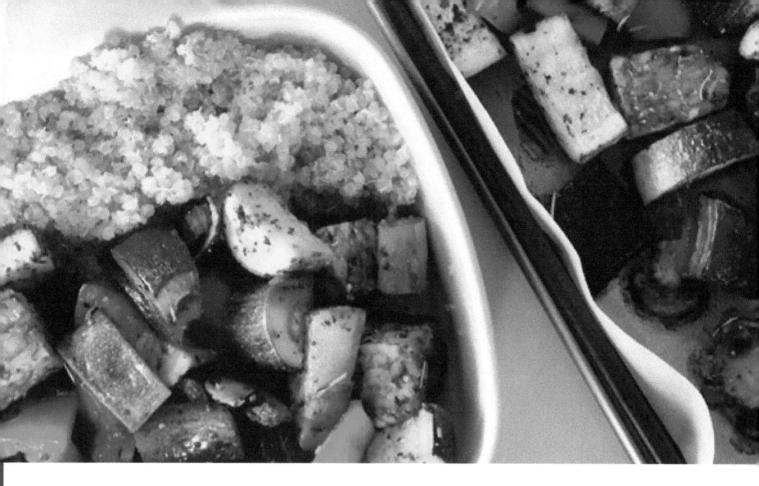

ROASTED BALSAMIC TEMPEH WITH VEGGIES

Training Day

Yield: 4 servings

Total Time: 30-35 minutes

Ingredients

(All veggies chopped into 1" pieces):

- 2 red bell peppers
- 2 carrots
- 2 zucchinis or squash
- 1 red onion
- 2 cups button mushrooms

- 1 package organic tempeh
- 3 tablespoons balsamic vinegar
- 2 tablespoons extra virgin olive oil
- ½ teaspoon sea salt
- ½ teaspoon pepper

Directions

1. Preheat oven to 425F. Line a large baking sheet with parchment paper.
2. Add the vegetables and tempeh to a large mixing bowl, then pour balsamic vinegar, olive oil and italian seasoning over the top. Toss to combine.
3. Transfer the veggies and tempeh to the baking sheet and roast for 25 to 30 minutes until the vegetables are tender and tempeh has browned.
4. Remove from the oven and pair with cooked quinoa or cauliflower rice.

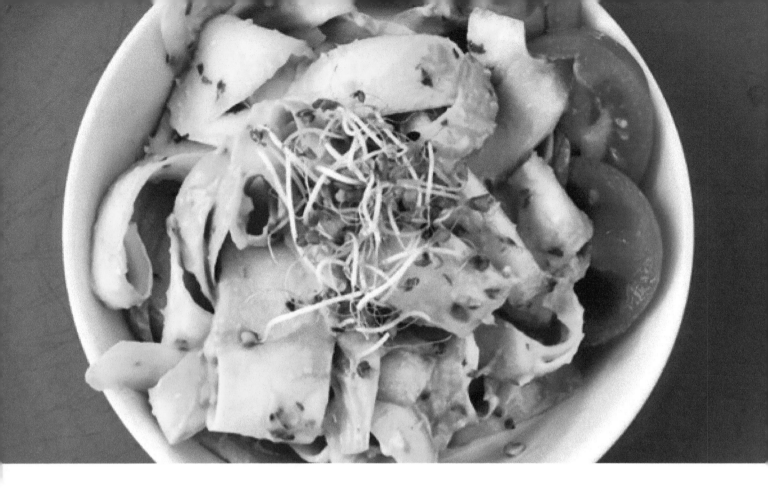

CREAMY AVOCADO ZOODLES

Rest Day

Yield: 4 servings

Total Time: 5 minutes

Ingredients

- 2 medium Haas avocados (ripe, seeded and peeled)
- ½ cup fresh basil leaves
- juice of 1 lemon

- 2 tablespoons minced garlic
- 2 tablespoons extra virgin olive oil
- sea salt and pepper to taste
- 2 medium zucchinis, spiralized or peeled

Toppings

- Cherry tomatoes
- Walnuts

- Broccoli sprouts

Directions

1. Add all ingredients (minus the zucchini) into a food processor. Set processor on low and run it until the mixture becomes smooth and creamy. Scape down the sides as needed.
2. When ready to serve, add a portion of the creamy avocado to the spiralized zucchini. May be used as a condiment or dressing for salads.
3. Store leftover avocado cream in an airtight container in the refrigerator up to 3 days.

Pro-tip: Keep avocado fresh by placing a raw onion in the container.

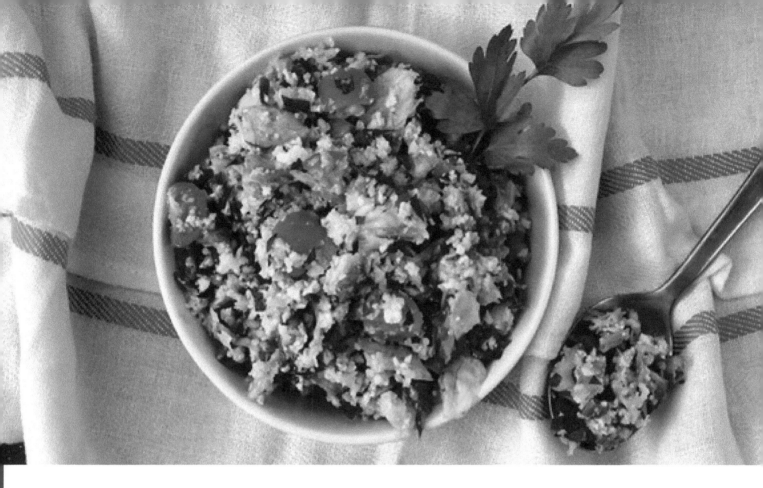

CAULIFLOWER TABBOULEH

Rest Day

Yield: 4 - 6 servings

Total Time: 10 minutes (not including "rest" time)

Ingredients

....

- 1 large head cauliflower, grated
- ¼ cup green onions, chopped
- ½ cup cherry tomatoes, halved
- 1 cup romaine, chopped
- ½ to 1 cup fresh parsley, chopped

- juice of 1 small lemon
- 1 tablespoon minced garlic
- 3 tablespoons extra-virgin olive oil
- sea salt and pepper, to taste

Directions

....

1. In a large mixing bowl, combine the cauliflower, green onions, tomatoes, romaine and parsley.
2. In a small mixing bowl, whisk together the remaining ingredients. Pour the dressing over the vegetable mixture and toss until well combined.
3. Cover and refrigerate for at least 30 minutes before serving. Salad can be stored in an airtight container in the refrigerator up to 3 days.

Pro-tip: Kick up the protein by adding scrambled eggs or ground turkey.

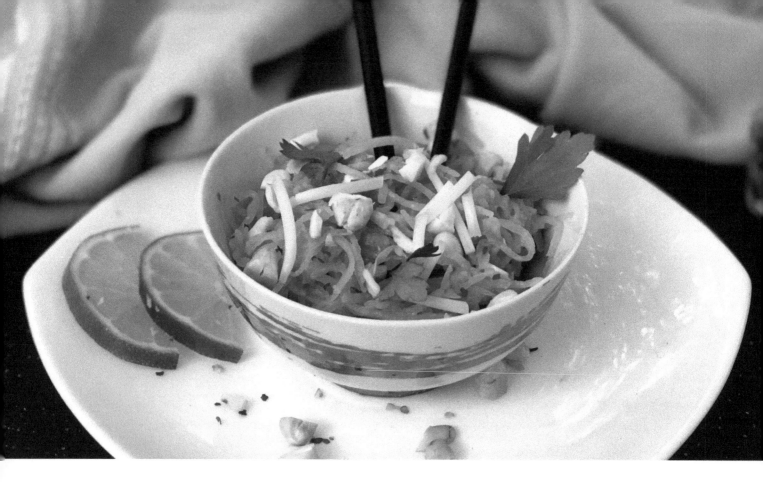

SPAGHETTI SQUASH
PAD THAI

....

Yield: 4 servings

Total Time: 45 - 50 minutes

Ingredients

- 1 spaghetti squash
- 1 tablespoon avocado oil
- ½ teaspoon sea salt
- ¼ teaspoon pepper

- 8 ounces cooked chicken breast or shrimp - optional
- 1 to 2 eggs

Sauce

- 2 tablespoons coconut aminos
- 2 tablespoon rice wine vinegar
- 1 tablespoon natural creamy peanut, almond or cashew butter
- 1 tablespoon coconut sugar - optional

- 2 teaspoons red boat fish sauce
- 1 teaspoon minced garlic
- juice of ½ lime
- pinch of red chili flakes

Toppings

- Bean sprouts
- Peanuts or cashews, chopped

- Green onions

Squash Directions

....

1. Preheat oven to 425 F.
2. Use caution when cutting the squash. Slice the ends off the squash and discard. Then, cut about 1 1/2" wide rounds of the squash. You can usually make 4 cuts in a small squash.
3. Set on a baking sheet lined with parchment paper. Use a fork to scrape out the seeds. Lightly drizzle with avocado oil and add salt and pepper.
4. Bake until the strands are tender but not mushy, about 30-35 minutes. If you prefer your spaghetti squash firmer, reduce baking time to about 40 minutes. Use a fork to pull the strands into the center of each round.

Pad Thai Directions

....

1. In a mixing bowl, combine all the sauce ingredients and whisk until smooth. Set aside.
2. Heat a non-stick skillet on medium, crack the eggs and cook until they are scrambled. Remove and set aside.
3. Pour the prepared sauce into the same skillet and bring to simmer for about 1 minutes. Add in the cooked squash noodles and gently combine until the sauce has been absorbed. (Option to add the sauce upon serving). At this time, add in the scrambled eggs and optional protein of choice. Toss to coat.

Breakfast

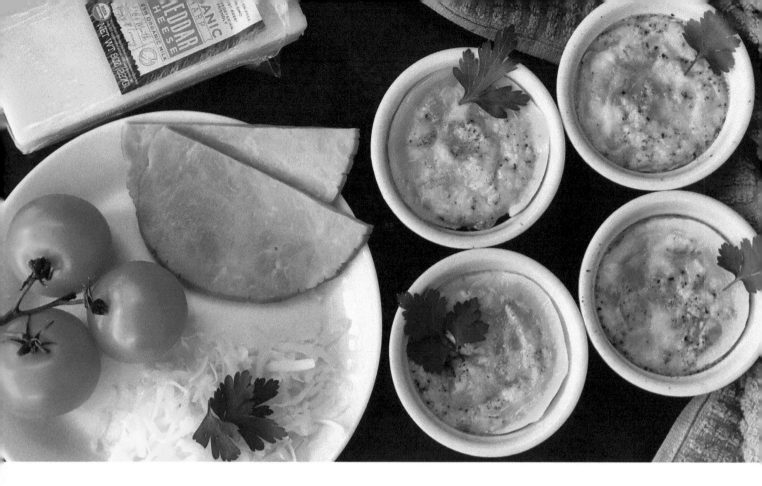

BAKED HAM & EGGS

Rest Day

....

Yield: 4 servings

Total Time: 25-30 minutes

Ingredients

- olive oil spray
- 6 large eggs
- 2 – 3 ounces sliced ham, cut into small pieces
- 1/4 teaspoon sea salt
- 1/8 teaspoon pepper

Toppings

- Fresh herbs
- Tomatoes
- Cheddar cheese

Directions

1. Preheat the oven to 350 F. Lightly grease four 4-ounce ramekins.
2. In a medium mixing bowl, whisk the eggs, ham, salt and pepper until well combined. Using a 1/4 cup measurer, divide the egg mixture equally between the ramekins.
3. Place the ramekins on a baking sheet in the oven and bake for 18-20 minutes until the eggs have puffed up and are set in the center.
4. Top with fresh herbs, tomatoes or cheese.

   Pro-tip: Reduce the fat content by using liquid egg whites in lieu of whole eggs.

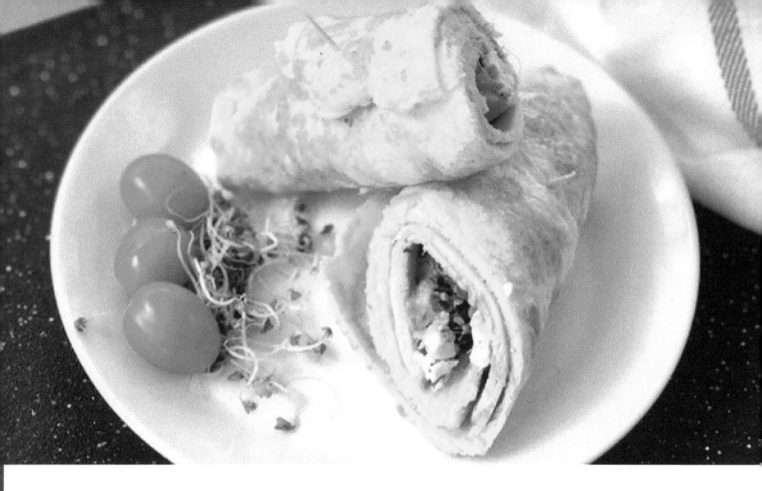

EASY EGG WRAPS

Rest Day

Yield: 1 servings

Total Time: 5-10 minutes

Ingredients

- 2 large eggs
- 1 tablespoon coconut flour
- 1 teaspoon baking powder

- pinch of sea salt
- 1 tablespoon coconut oil or grass-fed butter

Directions

1. In a medium mixing bowl, whisk the eggs until there are no lumps and you cannot see any egg yolk. Add the coconut flour and baking powder. Whisk until well combined and mixture is a smooth consistency.
2. Turn non-stick skillet to medium and add the coconut oil.
3. Pour the egg mixture into the skillet and rotate the pan to let the egg spread out into a thin layer. The thinner the better when using eggs as wraps.
4. Once cooked on one side, gently flip over with a spatula.
5. Remove the wrap and leave on a plate and allow to cool.
6. Repeat until you have made enough wraps for the week ahead.
7. Stuff with your favorite sandwich fillings and roll up.

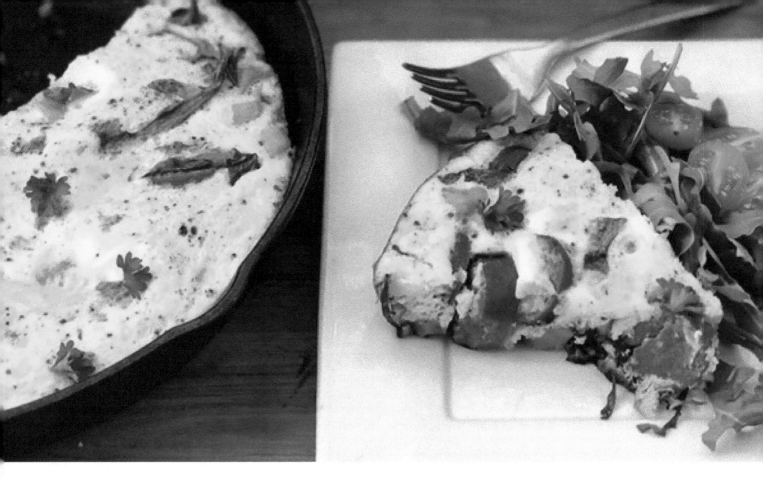

SKILLET FRITTATA

Training Day

Yield: 4 – 6 servings
Total Time: 25 – 30 minutes

Ingredients

- 8 – 10 eggs
- juice of 1 small ime
- sea salt and pepper, to taste
- olive oil cooking spray
- 1 tablespoon coconut oil, grass-fed butter or ghee
- 1 sweet potato, diced into small pieces
- 6 – 8 ounces (1/2 link) pre-cooked beef sausage or turkey sausage, sliced (optional)
- ½ red onion, diced
- 2 cups leafy greens

Directions

1. In a large mixing bowl, whisk the eggs until fully combined. Add the lime juice and season with salt and pepper. Set aside.
2. Heat a non-stick or cast iron skillet over medium-high heat. Spray skillet with cooking spray (this will help in easy removal of the frittata later). Add coconut oil/butter and allow to melt.
3. Add the diced sweet potato and sauté for 4-5 minutes. Season with salt and pepper.
4. Add in your sausage (optional) and onions. Continue to cook until the onions have slightly wilted and the sausage is warmed through. NOTE – You have the option of using any type uncooked ground meat, just make sure it is cooked through before you move to the next step.
5. Reduce the heat to low and add the greens. Gently stir and cook for about 2 minutes until they are just wilted. Sweet potatoes should be cooked through and tender now.
6. Spread everything evenly throughout the skillet and then pour the whisked eggs over the veggies and meat.
7. Cover the skillet and cook for 5-7 minutes until a light crust forms around the edge. The frittata should begin to pull away from the pan. (Meanwhile, turn broiler on low).
8. Transfer the frittata from the stovetop to the broiler and cook for 3-5 minutes until the center is set and top turns a golden color. Remove and allow to sit for a few minutes to cool down.

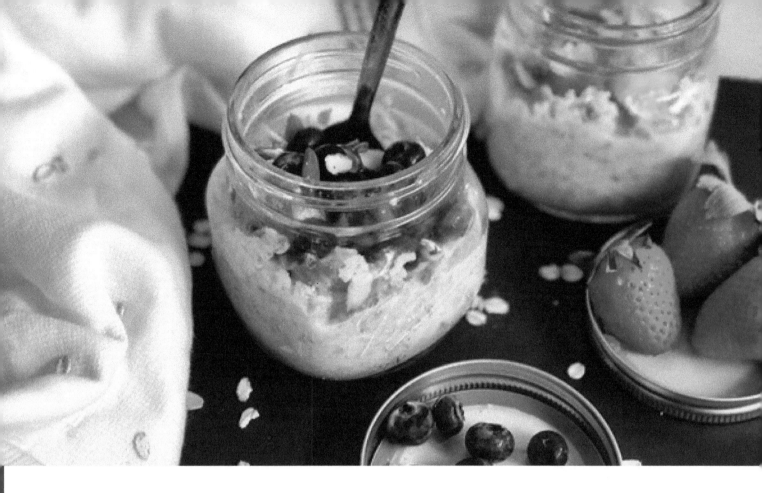

OVERNIGHT OATS

Training Day

Yield: 2 servings
Total Time: 3-5 minutes

Ingredients

....

- ½ cup rolled oats
- 1 cup unsweetened non-dairy milk (almond, cashew, coconut)
- 2 tablespoons nuts (walnuts, almonds)
- 1 teaspoon cinnamon or vanilla extract
- 1-2 teaspoons stevia or monk fruit

Optional:

- 1 tablespoon flaxseed meal
- ½ cup frozen or fresh fruit (strawberries, blueberries, raspberries)

Directions

....

1. Add all ingredients into a pint-size mason jar, screw the lid on top, shake and leave in the refrigerator overnight.
2. The next morning, add a dash or milk and microwave for 1 – 2 minutes. (Option to eat cold!). You can always little more sweetener if necessary.

Pro-tip: Make this a protein-packed breakfast by adding ¼ cup liquid egg whites or ½ a scoop of protein powder. Add more non-dairy milk or water accordingly.

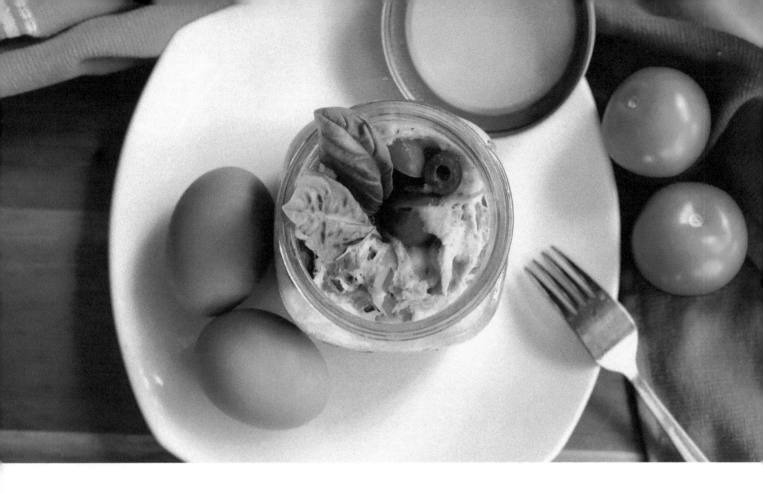

GREEK OMELETTE IN A JAR

Rest Day

Yield: 1 servings

Total Time: 10 minutes

Ingredients

....

- 2 large eggs
- ¼ medium red or white onion
- ¼ cup cherry tomatoes, sliced
- 3 tablespoons kalamata olives, pitted and sliced
- 2 tablespoons crumbled feta cheese

- 1/3 cup spinach leaves, thinly sliced
- 2 basil leaves, thinly sliced - optional
- ¼ teaspoon extra virgin olive oil or avocado oil
- pinch of sea salt and pepper

Directions

....

1. Add all ingredients to a 16-ounce wide mouth mason jar or pint-size jar. Secure the lid and leave in the refrigerator.
2. When ready to cook, shake until the mixture is well blended. Remove the lid and microwave for 1 ½ to 2 minutes until the omelet rises to the rim of the jar and there are no "liquidy" pools of egg. Carefully remove from the microwave and allow to cool for 5 minutes.

Pro-tip: Make this a training day meal by adding roasted sweet potatoes on the side.

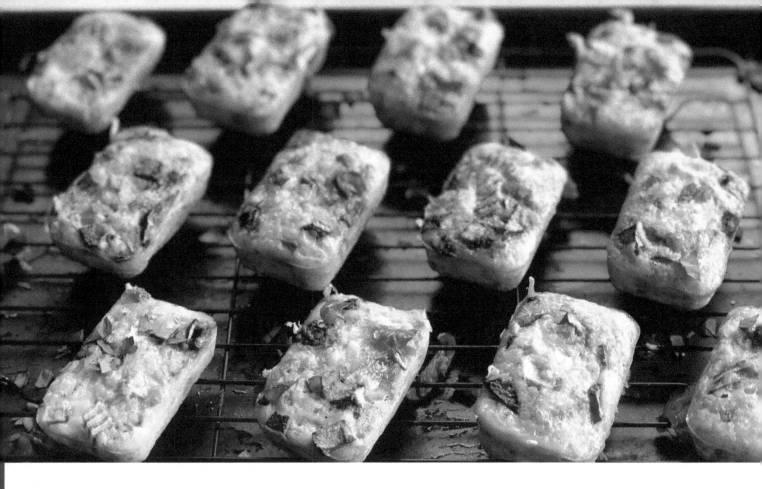

EGG & QUINOA BREAKFAST MUFFINS

Training Day

....

Yield: 12 servings

Total Time: 40 minutes

Ingredients

- 6 large eggs
- ¼ teaspoon sea salt
- ¼ teaspoon pepper
- 1 cup cooked quinoa

- ½ cup sundried tomatoes, chopped
- ½ small red onion, chopped
- 1 cup button mushrooms, chopped
- ¼ cup shredded parmesan or swiss cheese

Directions

1. Preheat oven to 350F.
2. In a large mixing bowl, whisk the eggs, salt and pepper.
3. Add the remaining ingredients and mix until well combined.
4. Spoon the egg mixture into a 12-count silicone muffin mold.
5. Bake for 22-25 minutes until eggs have fully set. (Insert a toothpick into the center and it should come out fully clean).

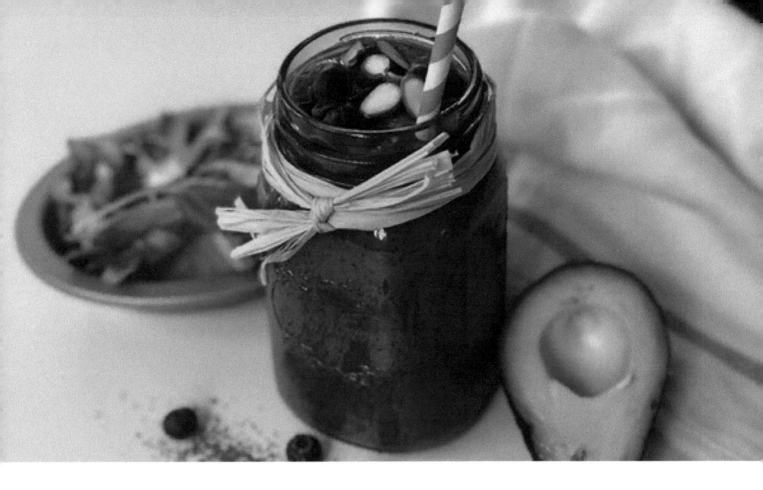

BLUEBERRY AVOCADO SMOOTHIE

Training Day

··

Yield: 2 servings

Total Time: 2 minutes

Ingredients

- 1 ½ cups unsweetened non-dairy milk (almond, cashew or coconut)
- 1 avocado
- 1 cup spinach
- ½ cup fresh or frozen blueberries

- 1 tablespoon ground flaxseed meal
- 1 tablespoon almond butter or sliced almonds
- 1 tablespoon granulated sweetener - optional
- ¼ teaspoon cinnamon
- 1 cup ice

Directions

1. Place all ingredients in a high-speed blender (in order).
2. For a thinner smoothie, just add more milk or water.

Pro-tip: Add collagen protein powder for hair, skin and nail benefits.

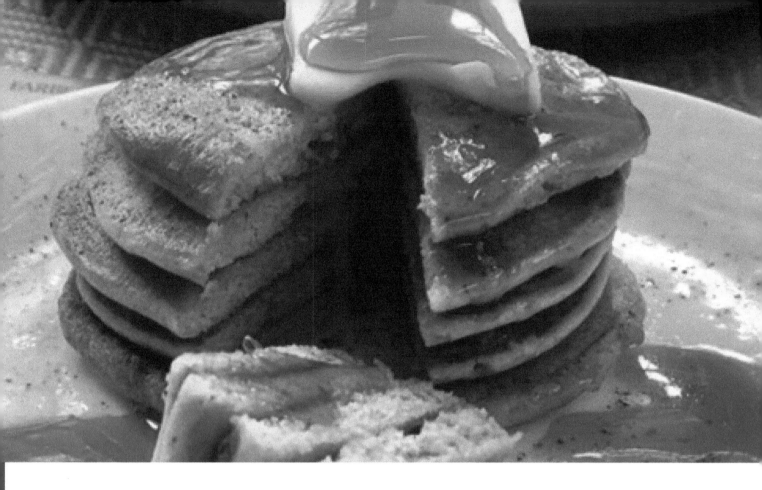

KETO PANCAKES

Rest Day

Yield: 4 – 6 servings

Total Time: 20 minutes

Ingredients

- 4 large eggs
- 1/2 cup cream cheese
- 1/2 cup almond flour
- 1/2 teaspoon cinnamon
- 2 tablespoons Swerve granulated sugar (optional)
- 1-2 tablespoons butter, ghee or coconut oil

Optional Toppings

- Blueberries
- Strawberries
- Cinnamon
- Lite maple syrup

Directions

1. Add all ingredients to a blender and mix until batter is smooth.
2. In a non-stick skill, over medium heat, add in the butter or oil.
3. Slowly pour in 2–3 tablespoons of batter per pancake and turn over once the center begins to bubble (usually takes about 3–4 minutes). You will have to do this in several batches so feel free to add more butter or oil to the skillet.
4. Once ready to serve, add toppings and compliment your pancake with eggs and bacon.

Pro-tip: For a dairy free version use Kite Hill almond cream cheese and coconut oil.

Desserts

Use the following recipes at your discretion and in moderation. Remember that desserts should be incorporated as "treats" on occasion, not every day. If you feel like you earned it, then have at it! Have ZERO guilt with these recipes as they contain quality ingredients.
.

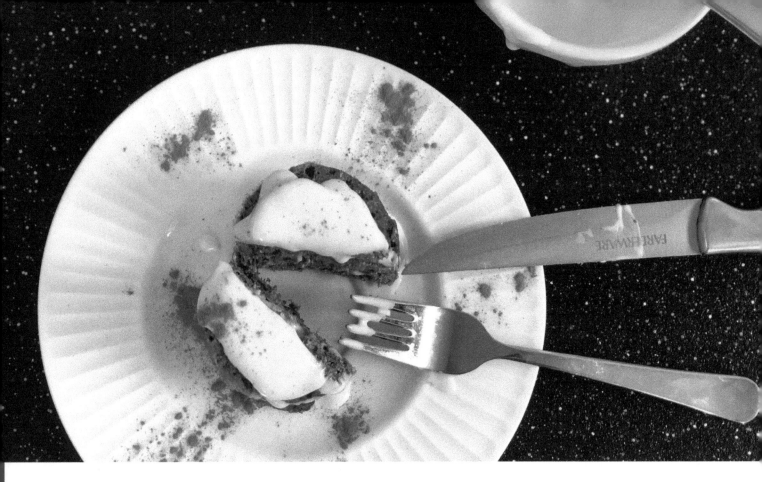

INDIVIDUAL MUG CAKE

....

Yield: 1 servings

Prep Time: 2 minutes

Ingredients

- 1 large egg
- 2 teaspoons coconut flour
- 1 teaspoon *Swerve* granulated sweetener
- 1 tablespoon unsweetened almond milk
- ¼ teaspoon cinnamon - optional
- 1/8 teaspoon baking soda

Toppings

- *So Delicious* Whipped Cream

Directions

1. Grease a microwave-safe coffee mug.
2. Add all ingredients and whisk until well combined.
3. Microwave for 1 to 1.5 minutes until the cake is set (done) in the middle.

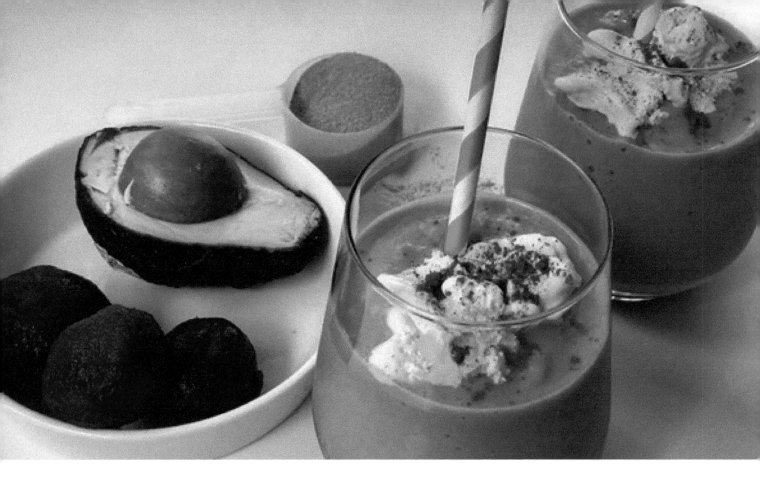

RED VELVET SMOOTHIE

Yield: 2 servings

Prep Time: 3-5 minutes

Ingredients

- 2 cups unsweetened non-dairy milk (almond, coconut or cashew)
- ½ avocado
- 1/3 cup Love Organic cooked beets or ½ small beet
- 3 tablespoons vegan chocolate protein powder or cocoa powder
- 3 packets *Monk Fruit in the Raw* or 2 tablespoons *Swerve* granulated sweetener
- ¼ teaspoon vanilla extract
- pinch of cinnamon
- 2 cups ice cubes

Topping

- *So Delicious* Whipped Cream

Directions

1. Add all ingredients (in order) to a high-speed blender and mix until completely smooth.

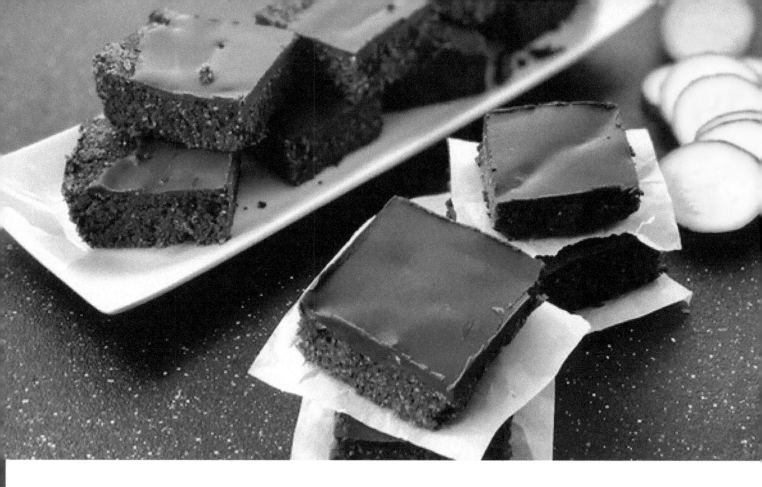

VEGAN ZUCCHINI BROWNIES

Yield: 16-20 servings

Prep Time: 30 minutes

Ingredients

- ½ cup zucchini (1 small), finely shredded and squeezed of excess water
- 1/3 cup coconut milk yogurt, almond milk yogurt or greek yogurt
- 1 cup + 2 tablespoons water
- ½ cup coconut oil, melted
- 3 tablespoons ground flaxseed/flaxseed meal
- 2 teaspoons vanilla extract
- 1 cup coconut flour
- ¾ cup cocoa powder, sifted
- ¾ cup *Swerve* granulated sweetener or xylitol
- ½ teaspoon sea salt
- ½ teaspoon baking soda
- ½ cup *Lily's* dark chocolate or *Enjoy Life* vegan dark chocolate chips
- ½ cup walnuts, chopped - optional

Frosting (optional)

- ¼ cup coconut oil, melted
- ¼ cup cocoa powder
- 1 tablespoon *Joseph's* lite maple syrup or *VitaFiber* prebiotic syrup

Directions

1. Preheat oven to 350F and line a 9 x 13 glass baking dish with parchment paper. Set aside.
2. In a large mixing bowl, combine the wet ingredients - zucchini, yogurt, water, coconut oil, flaxseed meal and vanilla. Mix well and let rest for at least 5 minutes.
3. In a separate mixing bowl, combine the remaining dry ingredients. Whisk until well combined. (If there are any clumps, simply use the base of a glass and press into the mixture to smooth it out). Pour this mixture into the large mixing bowl. Stir until even mixed. Consistency should be very thick.
4. Pour the batter into the baking dish and press down with a spatula or your fingers.
5. Bake for 19-20 minutes. Allow the brownies to cool for at least 15 minutes before cutting or adding the frosting. The batter will firm up as it sits and it will taste even better on the following day.

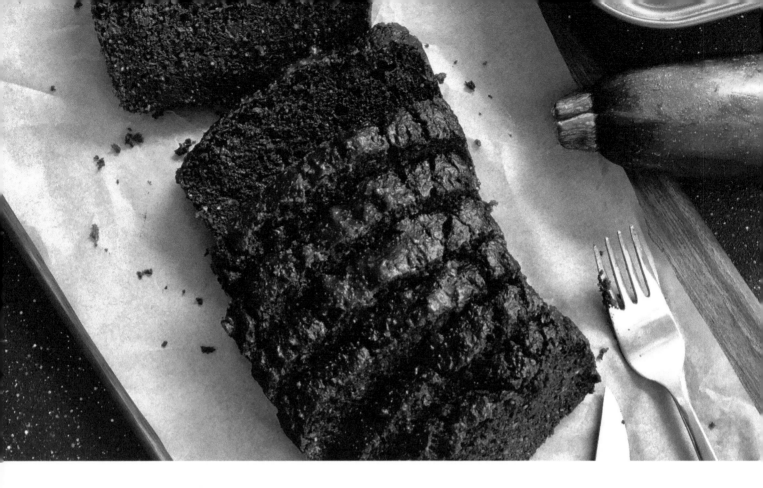

GRAIN FREE DOUBLE CHOCOLATE ZUCCHINI BREAD

....

Yield: 14 servings

Prep Time: One hour

Ingredients

- olive oil or coconut spray
- 2 medium zucchinis, grated
- ¾ cup + 1 tablespoon creamy peanut butter, unsalted
- ¼ cup *Joseph's* lite maple syrup or *Vitafiber*
- 2 whole eggs
- 1 teaspoon vanilla extract

- 3 tablespoons cocoa powder
- 2 tablespoons coconut flour or oat flour
- 1 teaspoon cinnamon
- 1 teaspoon baking soda
- 1 /4 teaspoon sea salt
- 1/3 cup *Lily's* dark chocolate or *Enjoy Life* vegan dark chocolate chips

Directions

1. Preheat oven to 350 F and grease a mini loaf pan with nonstick cooking spray. Your bread will turn out more like the shape of "biscotti" if you use a regular loaf pan.
2. Remove moisture from the zucchini by wrapping it up into paper towels or a dish cloth. Ring the excess water out so that the zucchini is not dripping, but so that it is still moist.
3. Transfer the zucchini into the large bowl and add the peanut butter, maple syrup, eggs and vanilla. Whisk until well combined and creamy.
4. Stir in cocoa powder, coconut flour, cinnamon, baking soda and salt. Mix until well combined.
5. Fold in the chocolate chips, reserving about a tablespoon for sprinkling on top.
6. Pour the batter into your greased loaf pan and smooth it over with the back of a spoon or spatula. Top with the remaining tablespoon of chocolate chips.
7. Bake for 40-45 minutes or until a toothpick comes out clean.
8. Once done baking, remove from oven and let it rest for 10-15 minutes. Once cool enough, remove bread from pan and transfer to wire rack to cool completely. Cut into 12-14 slices.

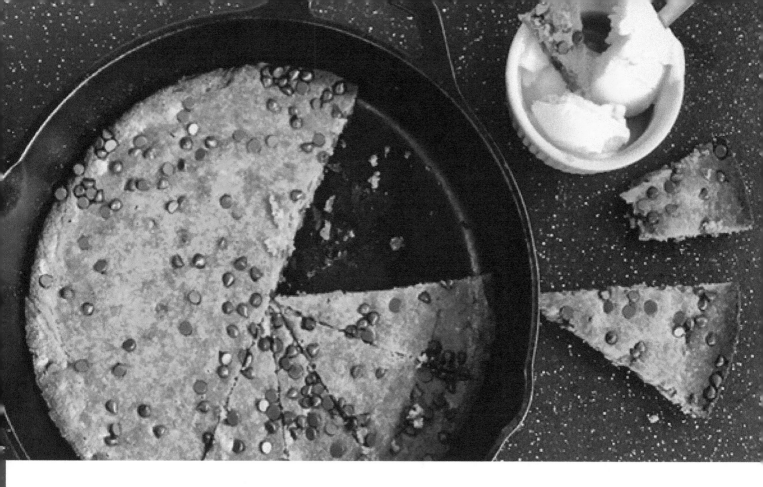

SKILLET CHOCOLATE CHIP COOKIE

Yield: 10-12 servings

Total Time: 25-30 minutes

Ingredients

- 8 tablespoons (1/2 cup) grassfed butter or ghee
- 1 large egg
- 1 teaspoon pure vanilla extract
- 2 tablespoons coconut sugar
- 1/4 cup *Swerve* granulated sweetener
- 2 cups super fine almond flour
- 1/2 teaspoon sea salt
- 1/3 cup *Lily's* dark chocolate or *Enjoy Life* vegan chocolate chips, divided

Directions

1. Preheat oven to 176C | 350F. Heat the butter in a 9-inch cast iron skillet over high heat until bubbling. Reduce heat to low and continue to cook while stirring occasionally until the butter begins to brown. A splatter screen may be beneficial here. Once browned, remove from heat and allow to cool for about 4-5 minutes.
2. While the butter is browning, whisk together the egg and vanilla extract in a medium mixing bowl. Add the sugar and sweetener and whisk again until combined. Add the butter (once it has cooled) and mix well.
3. Add in the almond flour (pressing down on any clumps). Add the salt and half the chocolate chips. Gently until the batter is well combined and creamy. It may not be as thick as cookie dough. Spoon the batter back into the cast iron skillet and top with remaining chocolate chips.
4. Bake for 25-28 minutes until the edges start to brown or insert a toothpick into the center. Toothpick should come out clean.

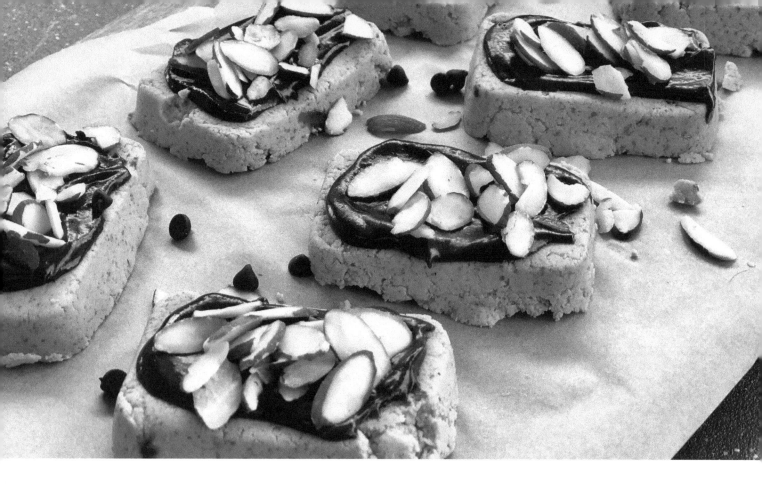

VEGAN PROTEIN BARS

....

Yield: 12 servings

Total Time: 25-30 minutes

Ingredients

- ½ cup creamy almond butter or peanut butter, unsalted
- 1/3 cup coconut oil
- ½ cup unsweetened non-dairy milk (almond/
- rice/cashew)
- 1 ½ cups vanilla or chocolate plant-based protein powder 1/3 cup almond meal1/3 cup almond meal

Optional Toppings

- 2 tablespoons *Lily's* dark chocolate or *Enjoy Life* vegan chocolate chips
- 1 tablespoon coconut oil
- 3 tablespoons almond slivers

Directions

1. In a medium microwave-safe bowl, combine almond butter, coconut oil and milk. Microwave in 30 second intervals until everything has melted. Make sure to stir in between and mix until well combined.
2. Add the plant-based protein powder (do not use whey powder) and almond and mix until mixture is well combined. This may take a few minutes as the dough will become thick and crumbly.
3. Use a 12 ct. silicone baking mold or line an 8 x 8" baking dish with parchment paper. Fill with the prepared dough and flatten out with your hands to make sure the dough is even. Place in the freezer for 5 – 10 minutes so dough can harden.
4. If adding the chocolate topping, combine the chocolate and coconut oil in a small microwave-safe bowl. Microwave in 30 second increments or until the chocolate has melted. Stir well. Pour over the bars. If you are using the baking dish, you may have to tilt the dish until all the bars are evenly coated. And if you are using the silicone mold, carefully remove each bar and pour the chocolate one-by-one. Top with slivered almonds and place back in the freezer for up to 20 minutes until chocolate has hardened.
5. Baking dish – remove from the dish by holding on the parchment flaps and place on a cutting board. Cut into 12 bars. Keep refrigerated in an airtight container up to 5 days or keep in the freezer for up to 2 months.

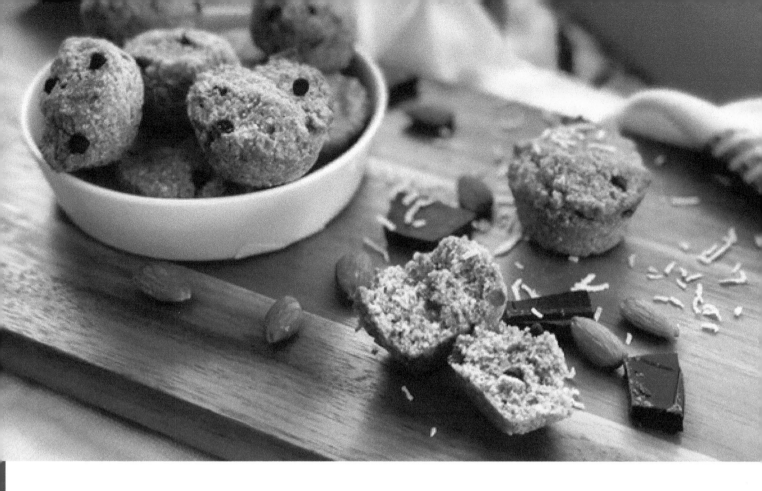

LOW CARB CHOCOLATE COCONUT BITES

Yield: 12 servings

Total Time: 20-25 minutes

Ingredients

- 6 tablespoons almond butter
- 2 whole eggs
- 1 teaspoon vanilla
- 5 tablespoons *Swerve* granulated sweetener or Xylitol
- ¼ cup coconut flour
- 2 tablespoons unsweetened coconut flakes
- ½ teaspoon baking powder
- ¼ teaspoon sea salt
- 2 tablespoons *Lily's* dark chocolate or *Enjoy Life* vegan dark chocolate chips

Directions

1. Preheat oven to 350F.
2. Combine the almond butter, eggs, vanilla extract and sweetener into a large mixing bowl. Use a hand mixer or fork to mix.
3. Add the coconut flour, coconut flakes, baking powder and salt. Mix until well combined.
4. Evenly distribute the batter into all 12 molds and bake for 15-17 minutes.
5. Allow to cool for 15 – 20 minutes before serving.

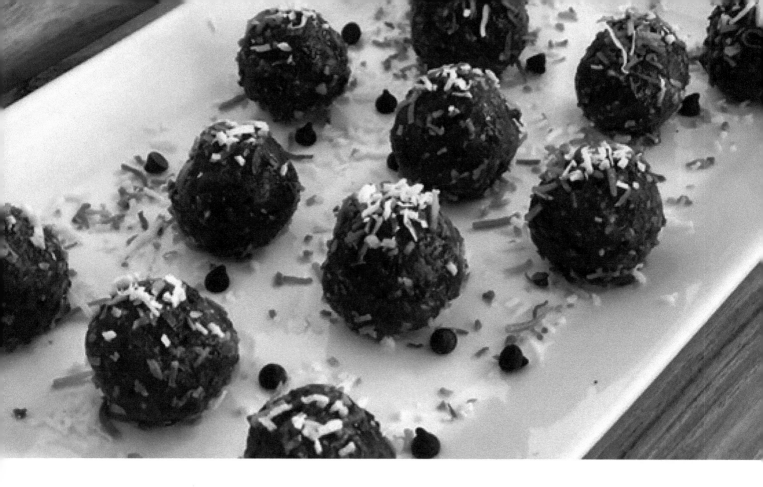

SAMOA COCONUT BITES

Yield: *12 servings*

Total Time: *30 minutes*

Ingredients

- 1 cup pitted dates (10), diced
- 1 tablespoon creamy almond butter
- 2/3 cup unsweetened coconut, divided
- 2 tablespoons *Lily's* dark chocolate or *Enjoy Life* vegan dark chocolate chips, divided

- 1/8 teaspoon vanilla extract
- 1/8 teaspoon sea salt

Directions

1. Preheat oven to 400 F. Spread all the coconut onto a baking sheet. Toast for 3 – 5 minutes until golden brown in color. Be careful not to burn the flakes.
2. Add the dates, almond butter, ½ of the toasted coconut, chocolate chips, vanilla and salt to a food processor. Pulse until the mixture becomes like a crumbly dough.
3. Using a cookie scoop, form 12 small balls. Then roll the balls in the remaining toasted coconut.
4. Store in an airtight container in the refrigerator for 3-5 days.

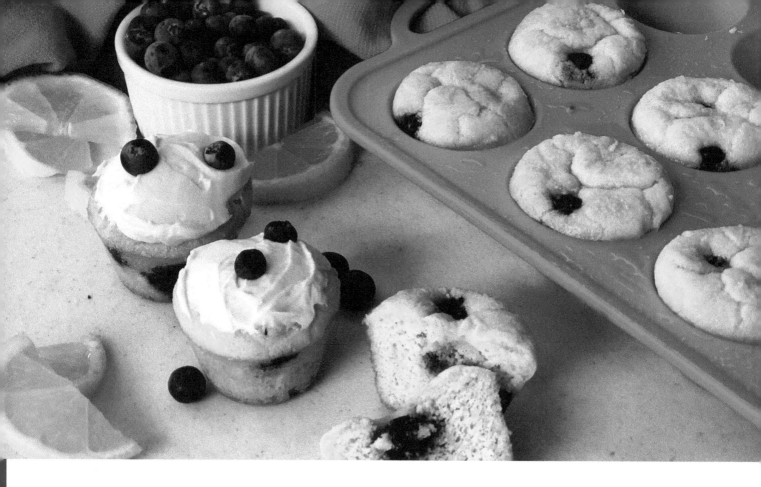

LEMON BLUEBERRY MUFFINS

Yield: 14-15 servings

Prep Time: 25 minutes

Ingredients

- 2 cups almond flour
- 1 cup heavy cream
- 2 large eggs
- 2 tablespoons butter, melted
- 5 packets (3 teaspoons) *Monk fruit in the Raw* or stevia

- 1/2 teaspoon baking soda
- 3/4 teaspoon lemon extract
- Zest of 1 lemon
- 1/4 teaspoon sea salt
- 3 ounces blueberries

Directions

1. Pre-heat oven to 350 F.
2. Prepare 2 silicone 12-count muffin tins. Note – add liners and coat with coconut spray if not using silicone.
3. In a large mixing bowl, combine almond flour and heavy cream.
4. Add one egg at a time, and stir until well combined.
5. Add the butter, sweetener, baking soda, lemon extract, lemon zest and salt. Mix well.
6. Fold in the blueberries and stir until they are evenly distributed.
7. Using a cookie scoop, fill each muffin to about 1/2 full.
8. Bake for 20 minutes or until edges are golden brown. Let cool and serve.

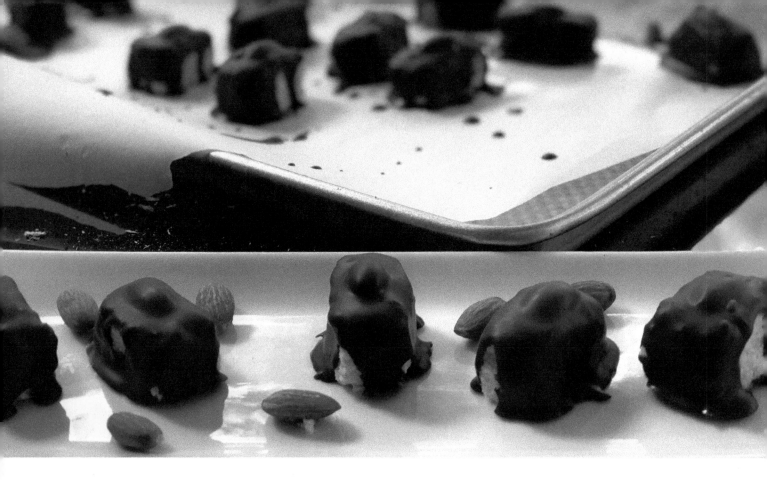

ALMOND JOY BITES

Yield: 20 servings
Total Time: 35 – 40 minutes

Ingredients

- 2 1/2 cups unsweetened shredded coconut flakes
- 1/4 cup *Joseph's* lite maple syrup or *Vitafiber*
- 1 teaspoon vanilla extract
- 1 tablespoon coconut butter - optional

- 1 ounce raw almonds
- 1 cup *Lily's* dark chocolate or *Enjoy Life* vegan dark chocolate chips
- 3 tablespoons coconut oil

Directions

1. Add shredded coconut, vanilla and maple syrup to a food processor and blend until coconut is moist.
2. Using a cookie scoop, roll into balls (or shape into ovals).
3. Place on parchment paper and add one almond to the top of each bite.
4. Place in the freezer for 15-20 minutes to allow bites to harden.
5. In a microwave-safe bowl, melt the coconut oil and then add 1 cup chocolate chips. Continue to microwave until mixture is smooth.
6. Spoon chocolate mixture over each bite. A fork can be used to hold the bite and prevent sticky fingers.
7. Repeat for each bite, then refrigerate for about 10 minutes so the chocolate can harden.

Take-away Tips

Do:

- Embrace a lifestyle change and shift your focus to overall health.

- Be aware and mindful of your daily habits by journaling.

- Enjoy "treats" on occasion with zero guilt

- Take progress photos and measurements every month.

- Experiment with different foods to optimize nutrient intake.

- Expect your journey to be anything but linear.

- Plan your days in advance.

- Embrace progress, not perfection.

- Exercise regularly, meditate, and be kind to your body.

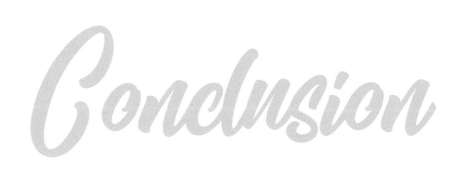

Conclusion

"The way to get started is to quit talking and begin doing."

Walt Disney

What's Next...

Start small

Start with small changes with your nutrition and exercise habits. The minute you shift your focus to a single action and not the end result; this is when you can truly transform. Micro goals lead to the Macro goal!

Be active

Exercise shouldn't be torturous (at least not every day). Find an activity that leaves you feeling accomplished. That means it has to be somewhat challenging. So get out of your comfort zone for just a few minutes!

Commit to at least 30 days

If you want this lifestyle to stick, choose one to two habits that you can commit to doing every single day. Whether it's a healthy tip from me or you want to focus on your water intake, stick to it consistently for at least thirty days. After you have set the habit, then you can then move on to the next set of habits and repeat.

Get family involved

Support and accountability from your loved ones is essential. Be active together, cook meals with each other and even create a family "goal" board.

Keep a Journal

This will help you remember how awesome you feel when you are sticking to healthier habits. Journaling can be an eye-opening experience especially if have never tracked your food or calories. It can also help you get a feel for portion control. So there's nothing to fear here. You can easily download free online trackers like My Fitness Pal or My Plate Counter.

The turtle always wins the race

Fast results are always tempting, but health should never have an end date. This journey should become a part of who you are and should eventually turn into a habit like brushing your teeth.

Want to find out more?

Get 150+ Free & Tasty recipes - just visit www.ninanyiri.com

Listen and learn as I provide helpful tips on the 4U Fitness Podcast.

Topics include:

- Carb Cycling
- Intermittent Fasting
- Dining out Recommendations
- Benefits of Sleep
- Reasons to Stay off the Scale
- Interviews with Successful clients
- Body Positivity & Self Care
- Protein Recommendations
- Cortisol Health

For Apple products:
https://itunes.apple.com/us/podcast/4u-fitness-podcast/id1258694711?mt=2

For Android products:
https://play.google.com/music/listen#/ps/Igl7s6wfwrj6xsa35h7c7ymy4du

Follow me on:
- Instagram @Nina_Nyiri & @4ufitnessllc
- Facebook @Nina Raquel Nyiri, 4U Fitness Personal Trainer
- Youtube @4U Fitness

If you are ready to start looking and feeling better, we have five beautiful fitness centers conveniently located in Tampa, St. Petersburg, Orlando, Boca, and Fort Lauderdale Florida.

Please email inquiries to: nina@4u-fitness.com or daniel@4u-fitness.com

Our mission:

Our purpose is to teach the population on how to exercise and build sustainable, healthy habits; thus changing the mentality of what it takes to be strong and healthy for a long and happy life. We are genuinely interested in educating our clients, so they can learn how to maintain and keep their results forever. The knowledge we have is not ours to keep and we will not compromise our ethics or integrity in the name of profits. By getting the results they desperately need and desire, our clients will gain back years to their lives.

About the Author

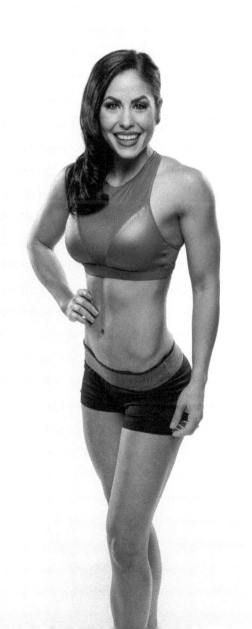

Nina and her husband Daniel run a thriving personal training business and their clients have had extreme success with life-changing transformations thanks to their unique approach to coaching. Nina holds a Master's Degree of Exercise Sport & Science from Texas State University, a B.S of Sports Management from Texas A&M University-Corpus Christi and Personal Training Certification among other accolades.

Nina believes that in order to achieve long-lasting results, certain habits need to be in order. And because each client is so different than the next, much flexibility, empathy, openness and understanding are necessary to help them grasp a healthier and new lifestyle. Instead of forcing them into extreme and sudden changes, she encourages clients to think about how the healthy habits can fit into their lifestyle so that way the experience is enjoyable not isolating.

She truly understands the connection between food and how it impacts our health. So it is her mission to help clients build a habit of home-cooking with simple and tasty recipes! Results are 90% nutrition so what we feed our bodies is vital to our success.

CPSIA information can be obtained
at www.ICGtesting.com
Printed in the USA
LVHW071340250319
611735LV00039B/740/P

9 780998 701714